Wall Pilates for Seniors

2 Books in 1

The Ultimate Guide to Improve Strength, Coordination, and Good Posture | 20 Minutes-Daily Full Body Workout

By

Emma Myers

Table of Contents

Book 1 Wall Pilates **6**

Introduction 6

Chapter 1: What is meant by Wall Pilates? **8**

1.1 Does Wall Pilates Work? 8

1.2 Pilates' Numerous Benefits for the Elderly 8

1.3 Tips for Seniors Looking to Start Pilates 16

1.4 The Foundational Concepts of Pilates 17

1.5 Questions & Answers 20

Chapter 2: How Pilates Can Improve Your Posture and Which Exercises Are Best **22**

2.1 How can Pilates help in correcting poor posture? 23

2.2 What Are the Most Effective Pilates Moves for Improving Posture? .. 25

2.3 How Much Time Does Pilates Take to Improve Posture? 27

Chapter 3: Pilates for injuries of Pelvic Floor muscles . 29

3.1 Why Do Pelvic Muscles Get Weak? 29

3.2 How Can I Tell If My Floor Muscles of Pelvis Are Weak? 30

3.3 How is Nervous System impacted by Pilates? 31

3.4 How practicing Pilates may assist the body's reaction to stress. 34

Chapter 4: Pilates and Chronic Conditions **36**

4.1 Research on Pilates' Usefulness in Pain of Low Back 36

4.2 The Correlation between Pilates& Parkinson's Disease 37

4.3 Pilates as treatment for arthritis 40

4.4 Is Pilates Risk-Free? 43

4.5 The advantages of Pilates for those with ongoing medical conditions . 43

4.6 Advice on Preventing Injuries for Senior Citizens 45

4.7 Modifications and Safety Measures to Take 46

Book Two 48

Workout and Stretching.. 48

Chapter 1: Stretching Before Pilates 49

1.1 How About Some Pre-Pilates Stretches?........................... 49

1.2 Full-Body Pilates Wall Exercise Example 54

Chapter 2: Pilates Exercises 61

2.1 Easy And Fun To Do Exercise 61

2.2 Wall Poses To treat Anxiety 75

2.3 Release Pain in Joints Using Pilates 79

2.4 Resistance Bands and Pilates...................................... 85

Chapter 3: 21-Day Workout Plan 96

.... 97

Conclusion...104

Book 1 Wall Pilates

Introduction

Joseph Pilates, the creator of Pilates, referred to his method as "Contrology" when he first introduced it to the world. This workout has been performed for more than 90 years but has only recently seen a boom in prominence. This is a one-of-a-kind workout for the full body since it employs motions that are regulated and perfect for helping you tone the entire body, enhance your posture, & increase flexibility while simultaneously strengthening the deep core muscles. In order to do a standard Pilates program, you will need to make use of specialist apparatus such as Wunda Chair, Reformer or Cadillac, all of which are commonplace in Pilate's studios. Because of this, doing Pilates exercises in the comfort of your own home is not the most convenient option, provided you have entry to a facility or are ready to make an investment in certain equipment. Wall Pilates, on the other hand, may provide an excellent exercise in Pilate's tradition without the use of any apparatus at all. Continue reading as we explain and walk you through a terrific Pilates exercise plan that you can do in the comfort of your own home.

Despite the fact that it has existed around for close to a century, Pilates is still growing in popularity and winning over new followers on a consistent basis. You may modify it to meet your needs and those of your health objectives, irrespective of the age, gender, current state of health, or current fitness level. This is one of the reasons why it has grown into such a prevalent form of physical activity.

Practicing Pilates may have a multitude of positive effects on a person's well-being, including enhanced flexibility, muscular tone, & strength. We addressed these advantages, as well as the many other elements of Pilates that contribute to the activity's overall value in this book.

As humans, we are prisoners of habit. We move in a particular manner, we take stairs in a particular way, we stand in particular way, and we also sit at our workstations a specific way. Therefore, due to excessive usage, our muscles become unbalanced. Pilates is a kind of exercise that helps to combat it.

Focus on each exercise, use of the muscles of abdomen & low back, flowing, accurate movement patterns, as well as controlled breathing are a few of the guiding principles of Pilates technique. Based on particular moves, Pilate's routines may be carried out on specialized devices, such as a bed-like frame known as a reformer, or they can be carried out simply against a wall.

Although Pilates represents strength training, it appears to be like majority of other exercises that go into that category that you are probably already acquainted with. The goal of Pilates is not so much to create muscle as it is to improve the tone of existing muscle, but ultimate effect is the same: increased stability & endurance. Pilates is not going to cause you to gain muscle mass; on the contrary, it will help you develop a longer and slimmer appearance. In spite of this, it is a good way to develop a solid physical basis for activities that involve increasing muscle, and it could even reduce the risk of injury.

You may discover that the study on health advantages of Pilates is more perplexing than it is beneficial if you look into it more. Contrary to that, there is a substantial body of research indicating that it may be beneficial to health of a broad variety of individuals and situations.

A century's worth of oral testimony (from individual's personal stories as opposed to study) ought not to be taken lightly.

Because of the possible advantages and typically minimal danger, it is well worth a try, much like tai chi, yoga, qigong, & other workouts that involve mindful movement. And similar to other forms of physical activity, the most critical considerations are whether or not you're fond of the activity and the way it renders you feel afterward.

Chapter 1: What is meant by Wall Pilates?

This form of Pilates employs body weight & resistance of wall to strengthen the muscles & increase the flexibility. It is a reformer type of Pilates.

This kind of exercise is perfect for newcomers to Pilates or those looking for a workout with little impact since it uses slow, controlled movements. You won't be concerned about the price or where to put any other equipment in the house since all you need is wall.

1.1 Does Wall Pilates Work?

The function of the wall is to provide the newcomer with a solid base on which to build. It provides a feeling of security and facilitates the attainment of more advanced poses.

Pilates at the wall might be a great place to begin for people who're new to exercise or are still recovering from injuries. Specifically, wall is helpful partner for resistance exercises, increasing the intensity of the workout and so facilitating the toning and sculpting of muscle tissue.

Wall Pilates has the potential to be a very effective workout if done correctly, providing all the same benefits as normal Pilates exercises.

1.2 Pilates' Numerous Benefits for the Elderly

If you're going to put in the effort to exercise, it's important to be certain your efforts are worthwhile. The benefits of Pilates are many. You'll also get a plethora of other advantages.

Strengthens the Core

Although most of us practice it, our bodies weren't designed to spend eight hours a day sitting on a chair. This might lead to weak abdominal muscles and poor posture. Pilates is a great way to combat this since it improves posture and fortifies abdominal muscles.

The muscles in back and sides, along with the ones in your abdomen, make up your core. The wall provides additional spinal support, making it easier for novices to focus on using their abdominal muscles during Pilates mat exercises.

In today's society, leading a life of inactivity is quite prevalent. Back discomfort is one of the symptoms that may result from spending the whole day seated at a computer and not getting enough exercise. In many cases, weakness in the core & poor posture can render this condition much worse.

Pilates performed against wall is an excellent method for improving posture & strengthening the abdominal muscles. When most people read the term "core," their first thought is of the muscles over stomach. However, "core" refers to all of muscles in the human body, including those in the back & sides.

When performing mat Pilates yourself, it might be challenging to focus on correctly activating your abdominal muscles, but wall provides additional support for the spine. This makes it possible for anyone to concentrate performing the exercises.

Increases flexibility

Pilates's appeal is partly due to the flexibility it renders you. Pilates, in contrast to typical training programs that promote muscular development, lengthens muscles in body, making you appear longer as well as thinner.

By offering stability and support, the wall may be utilized to assist you in deepening a stretch & increasing flexibility.

The typical weightlifter could have trouble touching their feet despite being capable of deadlifting almost twice their body weight. This was my condition up until I began making regular Pilates practice a part of my life.

It is commonly recognized that Pilates may improve agility while at the same time strengthening muscles. When doing exercises, you may improve your agility and range of movement by using the wall to help you achieve deeper stretches.

Pilates emphasizes both flexibility and strength. Pilates creator Joseph Pilates famously observed, "True agility can be attained only when every muscle is equally developed." The human body works like a set of levers & pulleys. However, we seldom use that strategy during a stretch as well as when we lift weights. In Pilates, however, such is not the case. Pilates' focus on the relationship between the mind and the body and its ability to rectify imbalances has revolutionized flexibility training industry.

Pilates helps the neurological system operate better because it activates the core muscles, which are often neglected in favor of more popular muscle groups. The nervous system sends a cascade of instructions from brain to such muscles when you first use them after they have been sleeping for decades. As a result of the "turning on" of neuromuscular networks, the brain feels like it has a greater handle over body. As we become older, this becomes more important if we want to keep our independence and dignity intact.

Strength and endurance of the muscles

Muscle endurance is an important attribute to have, especially as we age. Muscular endurance is essential for regular activities like grocery shopping & playing with kids since tired muscles would make these chores impossible. Better performance in gaming and other physically demanding activities is another benefit.

Pilates on the wall is a great way to work out since the slow, controlled movements are great for building muscular endurance. Constant physical exertion, such that caused by this, leads to greater endurance. The added muscle-building resistance from wall is a nice bonus.

Muscle endurance is much like any other aspect of fitness that depends heavily on the impact that a certain workout has on muscles. The term "muscle endurance" describes a muscle's or group of muscles' ability to contract repeatedly under constant resistance.

We often talk about the number of repetitions you can do in the gym or how long you can hold an activity such as planking. Muscular endurance, however, is a kind of functional fitness that is essential for things like childrearing and grocery shopping.

Muscle endurance and strength may be improved with the aid of Wall Pilates by engaging in slow, regulated sequences of motion as well as increasing "time under load" in the context of incremental overload. You may add "weight" to your exercises without actually using weights, thanks to the added resistance provided by the wall.

Low-impact workout

The force exerted on a person's joints during a certain action is referred to as "the impact." High-impact workouts like jogging as well as jump squats, may place a tremendous lot of strain on body, which can lead to aches and pains in the joints and other areas.

Low-impact workouts, such as Pilates, are great for maintaining physical fitness without putting undue strain on body's joints. Pilates is fantastic choice for anyone whose mobility is limited by joint pain or other issues.

Help Rehabilitation of the body

Due to low-impact character of this exercise and its ability to improve flexibility, muscular endurance, and core strength, Pilates is regularly used in physical rehabilitation procedures. Patients recovering from surgery, or an accident may find comfort in the wall's stability as well as support. It may also be a great way to help the body into some more advanced positions.

Pilates Increases Bone Density

While Pilates also has some unexpected bone-building advantages, exercising for strength is a well-known method for increasing bone density. "Bone, similar to muscle, adapts to weight-bearing and resistance exercises.

Muscles draw on bone during resistance training to produce tension, which strengthens the bone. Reformer springs &Pilates rings provide resistance in context of Pilates.

Pilates Burns the Calories

Pilates is a calorie-burning exercise, but it will not burn the same number of calories in same period of time as, for instance, jogging. In beginner's Pilates routine, you will burn 4 calories every minute, 6 calories every minute in middle-level routine, & eight calories every minute in advanced routine, according to data from the IDEA Health & Fitness Association.

Your actual calorie burn will obviously vary on the weight, degree of fitness, & intensity.

Pilates Reduces Back Pain

Pilates develops core to stabilize the back, encourages proper alignment, & provides mild stretching for stiff back muscles. Additionally, Pilates corrects structural abnormalities that often result in bad posture & back discomfort. Roll-up & swan prep are two specific Pilates moves for strengthening spine.

Core strength is improved with Pilates.

Working on one's abdominal muscles is an essential component of any Pilates session. Pilates is total-body workout; however, it's primarily focused on musculature of trunk and hips, dubbed Pilates powerhouse. Pilates is a workout that can be done anywhere.

Traditional crunches are not nearly as helpful as Pilates when it comes to strengthening the abdominal muscles, notably obliques. Pilates is centered on properly contracting the abdominal muscles during every exercise.

To provide just one example, during seated arm sequence on reformer, it's essential to keep the abdominal muscles contracted in order to keep the spine steady and properly perform exercise. Pilates places an emphasis on optimal alignment and appropriate form, which necessitates an active engagement of the abdominal muscles.

Pilates may be beneficial in reducing the risk of injury.

Pilates can help you become more flexible, it can help you get stronger, and it can help you become more balanced, all of which may lower the chance of injury. As you bend down to pick stuff up off the floor, there is a chance that you may injure your back. However, if you are able to enhance the flexibility of your hamstrings, this risk could be reduced. On the other side, increasing one's strength means better control of activity, which also reduces injury.

Pilates that is performed unilaterally (on 1 leg / one side) may help improve balance and lessen the likelihood of injury from falling. According to Gurka, Pilates promotes body awareness, which helps to generate efficient movement sequences, which in turn reduces the amount of stress placed on tendons, joints, muscles, & ligaments.

Since Pilates is gentle on the joints, it also does not require a great deal of cardiovascular fitness. You will be happier, healthier, and less prone to injury because of the emphasis on core strength and mind-body training to develop strength and flexibility. I went to Pilates studio and did a few lessons to help slow the growth of osteopenia, osteoporosis & arthritis. Pilates is particularly helpful for people with osteoarthritis & osteoporosis. Stronger muscles can support more of body's weight. The relief to the joints is, therefore, possible. Pilates has been shown in certain studies to mitigate the effects of osteopenia & osteoporosis. Physical therapists believe that the amount of benefits of Pilates is vast.

You'll find that your adaptability improves.

The vast majority of workouts simply involve mobility in one dimension at a time. And in most cases, that's the action of moving forward & backward (as in crunches). Pilates involves mobility in various dimensions.

Pilates workouts transfer spine between flexion and extension, internal rotation and external rotation, plus side bending, thereby increasing range of motion all over body. Engaging in activities that take place within these extra dimensions of motion develops and enhances flexibility while reducing the chance of injury.

Pilates is an excellent kind of cross-training for athletes.

Avoid putting yourself in danger of injuries caused by overuse by never altering up your training routine. Pilates is an excellent form of cross-training for joggers, particularly because stress generated by running is transferred through the core, & Pilates is an excellent workout for the core. Pilates additionally trains the entire range of movement of the hip joints that can improve both your stride & general jogging mechanics."

Pilates Betters Posture

Shoulders that are rounded and have bad posture are often the result of spending the entire day sitting at computer and staring at smartphone for long periods of time. The resulting muscle imbalances develop over time. Pilates helps counteract the consequences of these negative behaviors by generating improved muscular balance and symmetry.

Pilates encourages engaging a particular muscle once, separating muscles that may be less powerful, regaining any strength lost, and establishing balance throughout the body.

Building a solid core not only improves your posture but also makes it possible for you to effortlessly go through your everyday activities without experiencing any discomfort.

Knowledge of how to maintain the body correctly develops when the muscles responsible for maintaining it are exercised and strengthened.

It Increases Your Cardiovascular Capacity

As is the case with the majority of exercises, the intensity with which you perform Pilates determines the cardio advantages you get. Exercises in prone or sitting positions, such as seated twists & leg circles, tend to be inadequate in intensity for them to have a lot of impact on heart rate whatsoever. However, advanced maneuvers such as jack-knifing, in addition to side lifts, can be sufficiently strenuous to raise the heart rate to level that is well inside the goal zone.

You continue to be moving throughout a real mat routine, & it certainly qualifies as cardiovascular exercise at a moderate aerobic level. "Mat work is a great way to get in some light aerobic activity. Picture yourself walking up hill at a brisk pace or at steady pace."

If you want to improve your cardiovascular fitness, you should try to reduce the amount of time you spend recovering between activities and move swiftly between them. In high-intensity types of Pilates, you bounce from one exercise to another exercise quickly, which helps raise your pulse into aerobic zone. Building endurance requires maintaining a consistent effort throughout session.

Pilates Lowers Stress Levels

An effective Pilates practice ought to involve both high-intensity sections and soothing, mindful exercises that emphasize releasing tension. Breath principle" is the aspect of Pilates that offers the most benefit. By paying attention to linking the breath to the movement, you enable the CNS to drop, which has a soothing effect. There is a direct correlation between the two. You also develop the ability to inhale through unease, which may extend to stress control beyond the scope of the workouts."

Pilates might assist you in falling asleep.

The relaxing advantages of these activities may also lead to improved sleep. Research that was published in Bodywork & Movement Therapies journal found that formerly sedentary individuals who performed Pilates twice per week for period of twelve weeks noted improvements in quality of their sleep as well as their general life quality.

This could be due to the fact that Pilates permits one to concentrate on the here and now rather than dwelling on the difficulties of past or worries of future. Meditation may be practiced just by merely being in room; one need not be still or quiet in order to practice it. Taking the time out of our busy schedules to perform Pilates sessions allows us to regain our mental and physical equilibrium, which is helpful when we have a lot happening in our everyday lives.

Exercise with Little to No Impact

The impact of a task is force that is applied to the joints when you are participating in that activity. Running plus leaping have a larger effect on the joints & feet than other types of exercise, and they have the potential to create excessive joint discomfort. This is particularly true for persons who are new to exercising or are recovering from an accident. Low-impact workouts, such as stepping & walking, place less pressure on the joints and feet than high-impact exercises, such as running.

Because it is low-impact form of physical activity, wall Pilates is an excellent choice for those who suffer from joint discomfort or ailments that restrict their ability to move around. Due to its moderate impact, it is often used in rehabilitation programs because of its ability to develop agility, & muscular endurance.

People who are healing from injuries may lean on wall for assistance, and you may additionally utilize it to help ease your body into postures that are physically more demanding.

Alleviate pain and discomfort.

Pilates works to improve posture by building stronger leg muscles. Increased strength in these muscle groups shifts the body's weight away from the joints, reducing inflammation and discomfort. Pilates also provides a kind of meditation since it encourages concentration on the present moment and how one's body is feeling. There have been observable alterations in pain-related brain regions after practicing this kind of meditation.

Brain-body interaction

Pilates requires a lot of concentration since the motions are so subtle. In this training regimen, the mind is always engaged. You'll improve your flexibility, strength and coordination by training your mind and body to operate as one. This is the kind of physical activity that requires complete mental focus. The end outcome is a more optimistic state of mind. Investigators at Illinois University showed that those who practiced mindful exercises like Pilates had higher levels of brain activity. Pilate's exercises are similar in this regard since they call for intense concentration. And if that weren't enough, a recent piece in New York Times detailed the ways in which physical activity promotes new brain cell development while preserving existing cells in memory-related regions of brain. What could be better for mental arousal than purposeful physical activity?

Better breathing and less anxiety

Pilates places a premium on breathing since it aids in carrying out the exercises. You may lower your stress levels by training your mind and body to work together, specifically by learning to regulate your breathing. Furthermore, the kind of concentrated attention required by Pilates is a sort of mindfulness that has been shown to lessen inflammation while safeguarding against degenerative diseases like Alzheimer's.

Weight reduction

Pilates is great for weight reduction since so many of the movements focus on drawing the belly button toward the spine and holding that posture. Losing weight from your stomach won't result in washboard abs, but it will help your body seem more toned overall.

Pilates employs our own body weight to increase stamina, strength and endurance. As you compress and stimulate your muscles for correct alignment, support, & completion of the movements in Pilates, legs & arms will be "turned on" regardless of whether they are actively moving or not. Muscles toned & strengthened in this way have tremendous stamina & endurance.

1.3 Tips for Seniors Looking to Start Pilates

• Which clothing is appropriate: Put on some socks! Working out on a mat or piece of exercise equipment made of non-slip substance is good. Put on loose-fitting garments that nevertheless flatter your shape. Bottoms may be either yoga capris or regular trousers. On top, you may wear lightweight, breathable sports shirt. Don't wear anything that hangs freely off your body since you'll be moving about, and you do not want to worry about your clothing getting stuck on anything.

• Pilates etiquette: Since Pilates, like yoga, needs full attention from its practitioners, it is unpleasant to check your phone during a workout. Fix a time to get settled in and mute your phone.

• Drink water: Have a few glasses of water a couple of hours prior to session and another one within thirty minutes of the beginning of class to keep yourself hydrated. Drink little amounts of water as needed throughout session and down a full glass when it's over.

• Eat light: Consume a small snack before Pilates since some individuals find that performing yoga after a large meal causes them to experience nausea. Keep your pre-class eating to a minimum and focus on small snacks.

• Warm up: To make sure that your joints and muscles are flexible, it's important to first warm up. This aids in damage avoidance as well.

1.4 The Foundational Concepts of Pilates

Basic Pilates Concept 1: Breathing

Pilates uses breathing techniques to strengthen the link between brain and body. The objective is a steady, regular rhythm in one's breathing. This calls for a complete out breath and deep breath, both into belly instead of the chest.

In Pilates, you start each new movement with a deep breath. Activating the abdominal muscles & bolstering spinal stability is a common purpose for the exhale. The act of inhaling may be utilized to extend and relax the body.

Gains from Taking a Deep Breath:

Reduces Worry and Stress

It has been shown that slow, deep breathing helps reduce stress-related physiological responses such as heart rate & blood pressure.

Boosting Blood Flow

The circulation of oxygenated blood plus the elimination of waste products are both aided by deep breathing.

Pain Relief

When you breathe deeply, you may lessen muscular tension and discomfort.

Reducing Risk of Heart Disease

Cardiovascular system may be strengthened & heart health improved by practicing deep breathing techniques.

Basic Pilates Concept 2: Maintain Focus

Pilates requires complete mental focus. You need to pay 100% attention to the exercise and muscle area you're targeting. This ensures that you are working the right muscles and improving your form.

If you want to do a Pilates motion correctly, you should maintain your pelvis and shoulders relaxed while doing a leg swirl in the air. Isolating the right muscles and properly doing the exercise need mind-body links and focused attention.

As you aren't as prone to make errors while you are concentrating on the activity, you are less prone to get an injury.

The latest findings on mindfulness support the value of attentive focus in Pilates. Mindfulness meditation, which calls for intense focus, has been shown to help with a variety of health issues, including anxiety, hypertension, chronic pain, and poor sleep quality.

Basic Pilates Concept 3: Centre

Transverse abdominis are the "center" abdominal muscles. Rectus abdominis, long, flat muscle that helps bend the spine, is a part of this group.

• Abdominal obliques (internal & external) that help rotate the trunk and flex sideways are at sides of abdomen.

• The deep muscle layer that extends horizontally across abdomen & helps support the spine is called transverse abdominis.

• TVA is also known as "corset muscle" due to its role in providing support for the spine & waist. The transverse abdominal muscles are an important focus of Pilates exercises because of their role in core stability. Having a robust TVA is critical for spinal health and appropriate posture. It also aids in stomach flattening and producing a trimmer waistline. Activating the core (or finding your center) is a crucial part of Pilates. The abdominal muscles are targeted and strengthened throughout the workouts.

• People often think that TVA activation is same as just sucking in their stomach / bracing their abs. However, they are not the same thing at all.

Squeezing your abdominal muscles might make using your TVA more difficult. And tensing the abdominal muscles puts extra strain on back. Shallow breathing may be caused by overusing the abdominal muscles, which may result in their inhibition.

Activating the TVA muscles requires deep breathing. The diaphragm slides downward & contracts when air enters the lungs. By applying strain to stomach, TVA muscles are activated and strengthened via contraction.

Basic Pilates Concept 4: Maintaining Control

Joseph Pilates stressed the importance of being in charge. In his opinion, the quality of one's workouts was more crucial than number.

Pilates moves should be executed slowly and deliberately. This calls for deliberate, slow motion, with muscular effort taking precedence over momentum.

When you exercise deliberately, you put more emphasis on using the right muscles and avoiding injury. By reducing the likelihood of accidents, moving more slowly and deliberately may reduce the risk of harm.

It's normal to feel helpless in the face of one's body after years of inactivity, an accident, a sickness, or pregnancy. You may feel more at ease and in charge of the body again after engaging in Pilates.

You will learn how to utilize your muscles effectively and move the body in the most efficient manner possible. This will make normal, day-to-day movement less of a chore.

Having mental mastery is just as crucial as having physical control.

The ability to pay attention as well as be present in the present moment is essential for self-control. Focus is essential here. The brain will hone its ability to command your body's actions and movements with practice.

Basic Pilates Concept 5: Accuracy

Pilates also emphasizes the need for precision. The term "proper form" is used to describe whether an activity is carried out in the correct manner.

Learning the proper form for every Pilates exercise is essential when you're just getting started. This necessitates watching how you're standing and moving to make sure you're doing it properly.

You will improve your accuracy as you gain experience with the workouts. As a result, you'll be able to maximize the benefits of your workouts by focusing on the right muscles. You will be able to eliminate inefficient routines and improve your overall speed and agility.

Basic Pilates Concept 6: Flow

The ultimate aim of Pilates is to achieve effortless, flowing movement. "Flow" refers to this guiding concept.

Performing Pilates movements for the first time might seem unnatural and clumsy. Nothing unusual here! Correct form & muscle memory needed to execute the movements fluidly requires time to build up and develop.

Developing flow requires consistent practice and familiarity with exercises.

The workouts will become more fun and less like labor as your mobility improves. It might seem more like you are dancing than working out. It's hardly surprising that a majority of Joseph Pilates' first customers were ballerinas.

Improving your ability to "flow" will help you in many aspects of your life. The things that used to be difficult for you (climbing stairs, carrying groceries etc.) will become a breeze after you've mastered them.

Pilates' guiding principles are:

• Trusting one's gut and tuning in to one's body is essential.

• We may mentally rehearse the actions to improve our performance.

• The coordination of all muscles is our main concern.

• You shouldn't ignore any aspect of your body.

1.5 Questions & Answers

Here are some answers to the most common inquiries I get regarding the Pilates method.

What's the single most critical principle of Pilates?

While all tenets of Pilates are valuable, many believe that attention to breathing is paramount. Joseph Pilates thought that controlling one's breathing was the secret to maximizing the advantages of his exercises; thus, he emphasized it throughout all of his routines.

What are Pilates' three tenets of guiding?

Joseph Pilates, the creator of the Pilates method, founded his teachings on three pillars: (1) breathing, (2) entire-body health, & (3) total body devotion.

This suggests that he considered breathing to be an important part of Pilates and that he thought the practice could be used to enhance more than simply physical fitness.

The Pilates rule of control: what's the best way to explain it?

The capacity to move the body in a planned and deliberate manner is what we mean when we talk about control. Attention, diligence, and accuracy are needed here. Improve your command of your body and its movements with the aid of Pilates.

What are six fundamental principles of this exercise?

The six pillars of Pilates include focused breathing, a strong core, stable alignment, precise movement, and fluid transitions. To maximize the benefits of the Pilates routine, you must adhere to these guidelines.

What is the distinction between focus and accuracy?

Concentration is ability to pay close attention to one thing at a time and not let your thoughts wander. Precision means you're doing the moves the right way, with proper form & alignment.

To what end do we do Pilates?

Joseph Pilates created his workout method with the intention of boosting physical and mental wellness. Pilates is widely practiced today for its purported health benefits, including increased fitness, flexibility, & strength. However, the main objective of Pilates is to be able to move freely and easily (flow).

Does Pilates Require Good Balance?

No, balance isn't required, but it certainly helps. According to your current state of balance, there are a variety of adjustments that may be made to workouts to render them simpler or more difficult.

Chapter 2: How Pilates Can Improve Your Posture and Which Exercises Are Best

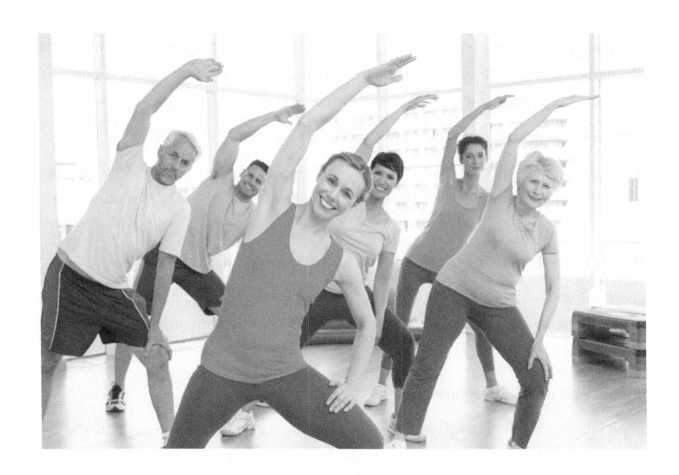

When your skeleton is in its proper place, the muscles are able to perform optimally, and the joints are spared unnecessary strain. The ability to take full, deep breaths is another benefit of good posture. On the contrary, slouching or slumping may cause muscular fatigue, joint discomfort, and limited motion. Does Pilates help with slouching? To put it simply, yeah. Pilates' primary purpose is to enhance both your movement efficiency & your coordination. Mastering to move from one's "powerhouse" or base is the primary goal. Powerhouse is region of body between pubic bone and navel. The benefits of learning how to employ core strength extend throughout the body but are most noticeable in the spine & posture.

2.1 How can Pilates help in correcting poor posture?

Pilates is great for improving alignment as well as posture because of its emphasis on core strength and flexibility.

Developing a healthy muscle length-tension relationship

There is an ideal duration at which each of your muscles contracts to maximize strength. The performance of a muscle decreases both when it is too short and when it is too long. The connection between length and tension is well-known.

Due to our sedentary lifestyles, length-tension connection of our muscles of posture is often disorganized.

The flexor muscles of hip (which connect to front of pelvis) might get shortened, for instance, if you hold a desk job & sit for extended periods. This may cause the lower part of the back to curve and the pelvis to lean forward, a condition known as anterior tilt of pelvis.

Another one is carrying one's head forward. Muscle imbalance, discomfort, and reduced range of motion are common consequences of forward-head stance, which is characterized by an anterior location of cervical spine.

By strengthening weaker muscles and extending the tighter ones, Pilates may help restore a healthy balance to body. As a result, your alignment and posture will improve.

Enhancing Stability of the Spine

Maintaining spinal stability is essential for proper posture. There are 33 vertebrae in spine, & each one is separated from its neighbor by a cushioning disc. Facet joints are tiny patches of cartilage that act as shock absorbers for the discs.

The ligaments and muscles around spine do their part to keep it in place. Instability in spine and slouching may result from a lack of or asymmetry among these muscles.

Pilates helps by building strength in muscles that support and stabilize the spine, which in turn may have a positive effect on one's posture & alignment.

Improving Flexibility in the Joints

Joint stiffness may develop from repetitive motions and poor posture. Because of this, you may find it difficult to move freely and upright.

Pilates helps increase flexibility in your joints, which makes it simpler to keep your spine in a neutral position.

Strengthening Your Core Muscles

Transverse abdominis plus pelvic floor muscles are part of the abdominal muscles lying deep that help keep the spine stable. Poor posture & pregnancy may both impair the muscles that help support your spine & pelvis.

Pilates is great for building core strength, which helps support your spine and pelvis. As a result, your alignment and posture may improve.

Teaching More Efficient Motion

Inefficient motion patterns can lead to poor posture. Pilates rehabilitates the body by re-educating it to operate in a more streamlined, controlled manner.

Pilates, with its emphasis on coordinated movement, is one method that has been shown to improve posture by retraining muscles in neck & shoulders.

When performed correctly, counter-extension exercises may retrain muscles of pelvis, spine and hips to improve posture.

Slow down the progression of deformity.

If you have poor posture and it is not rectified, you may develop a deformity. This is especially true with kyphosis (rounding of upper back) and lordosis (rounding of lower back).

Pilates' emphasis on proper form in movement has been shown to reduce the severity and rate of advancement of postural abnormalities.

2.2 What Are the Most Effective Pilates Moves for Improving Posture?

There are three main types of Pilates routines: those performed on the mat, on the Reformer, and on the Cadillac. Your posture may benefit from all three of these forms of exercise.

Pilates mat work is most basic form of the discipline and requires no special apparatus. These routines are often practiced on mat laid out on floor.

Reformer workouts are performed on a mobile platform. Reformer resistance may be used to strengthen and condition muscular tissue.

Cadillac exercises are performed on a big, stationary platform. People with ailments or problems with balance can benefit greatly from the Cadillac's support and stability.

Here are some Pilates moves that will help you improve posture:

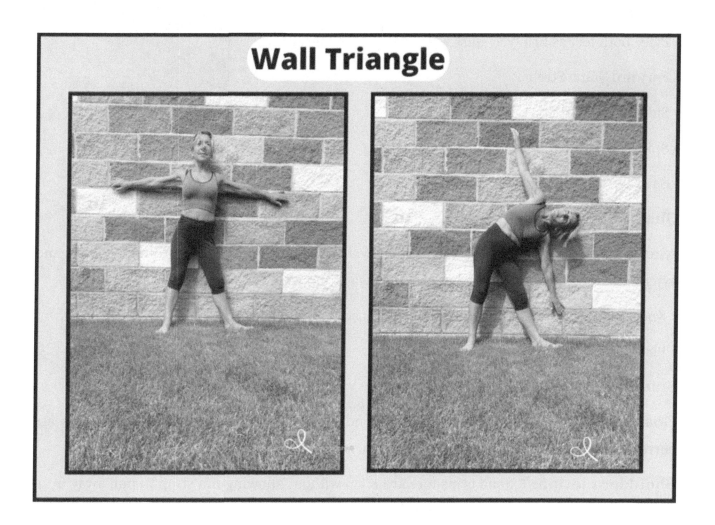

Wall Triangle

Wall Triangle

1. Place right heel against a wall while standing. Left leg should be externally rotated and positioned approximately two to three feet to side outwards, with left foot aligned to wall.

2. Ensure that both glutes are pressed up against wall. Place the head, shoulders, & hands on wall while extending the arms outward to T posture.

3. Keep your hands, shoulders and buttocks pressed against the wall while tilting your upper body as far to the left as possible.

4. To maintain this posture for between thirty seconds and one minute, contract your abdominal muscles.

Supine

• bridging with both feet up wall

• Seated

• Place both feet as firmly against wall as you can while sitting.

• Forward Spine Stretch

• Side-Lying

• Spine Twist

• Saw

Quadruped/Kneeling

• Step 1 foot back, stretch fully, placing foot level on wall with toes pointing directly down, and extend the other arm forward while looking away from wall. Go on to the same arm.

• Kneeling lunge with stretch of rectus femoris stretch: put back the shin up wall.

• Plank with your heels on wall

Standing

Goal Post: Extend arms straight ahead, bend elbows at 90 degrees to ensure fingers are currently pointing upwards, and gently open arms to wall.

Shoulder Flexion: Extend arms forward & up without allowing bra strap to pull away from wall. Without letting the bra strap detach from wall, try to contact wall with wrists.

• To roll down, start with feet about one foot farther from wall. As you slide down, progressively peel 1 vertebra at once away from wall. Roll upward gradually, segmentally moving through every vertebra. Move forward by bringing your feet near wall.

• Wall squat

• **Figure 4 stretch:** Leaning both buttocks onto wall

• Stand facing wall, raise one leg ahead, and put foot onto wall (strengthens standing glutes)

• Standing Scooter (push one foot onto wall facing inside the room, static hold)

The hundred

This workout aids in improving spine stability & abdominal muscular strength. Maintaining neutral spinal alignment while doing this exercise is crucial for maintaining healthy posture.

1. Stand with the arms at the sides & the legs in tabletop position. Your hips ought to be aligned with knees, and the knees ought to bend at 90 degrees.

2. Breathe out while you raise your neck, shoulders & head off mat. As you extend your arms in front of you while maintaining their level to the ground, inhale.

3. Count to 100 while exhaling and pumping arms up & down.

4. Throughout the workout, maintain a firm grip on your core and take deep breaths.

Legs out at an angle of 45 degrees

Now stretch your legs outward at an angle of 45 degrees so that tips of toes are in contact with the wall.

Touching wall will provide you with an additional bit of assistance for legs as you move along the exercise. Instead of lifting your head a few inches off the ground, try to lift your shoulders to the tips of your shoulder blades.

2.3 How Much Time Does Pilates Take to Improve Posture?

Improving one's posture is slow and steady process. Pilates works best when practiced on a consistent basis. It could take several weeks before you see a difference in your posture. Others may have to wait weeks, months, or longer.

The trick is to keep at it regularly and patiently. You'll be able to feel and see the improvements as the muscles become stronger and the posture straightens out.

Pilates isn't your only option if you want to see results quickly in terms of the posture. There are things like:

• Ensure that you're using seating that supports the back and maintains the spine in line if you devote a great deal of time working at a desk.

• High-heeled shoes, which may lead to slouched posture, should be avoided. Wear flats/shoes with minimal heels instead.

• Doing frequent physical activity: Be careful to supplement your Pilates with a regular fitness routine. Doing so can assist you in building muscle & straighten up your back.

• Maintaining an awareness of how you sit during the day. Keep your back straight, your shoulders back, and your posture upright.

• Misalignments in the spine may lead to poor posture, so getting regular adjustments from a chiropractor is a good idea. Correcting these errors and improving your posture requires frequent visits to chiropractor.

• You can improve your posture more quickly by doing all of these activities. However, maintaining a regular Pilates routine is crucial. You'll get there if you keep at it.

• Correcting poor posture with Pilates is an excellent goal. You may improve the posture and decrease your discomfort by working on your core strength along with the back muscles.

• Before beginning a new workout regimen, you should consult with your doctor/physical therapist. They can advise you on whether or not Pilates is a good fit for you and show you how it's done.

Chapter 3: Pilates for injuries of Pelvic Floor muscles

A collection of muscles known as pelvic floor / pelvic diaphragm "corset" around lower abdomen & hips. The bladder, uterus (if present), rectum, & bowel are all supported by these muscles. In addition to strengthening the muscles in core, they aid in keeping the pelvis in place.

3.1 Why Do Pelvic Muscles Get Weak?

Pregnancy and delivery are only two of many potential causes of weakened pelvic muscles. There are variety of workouts accessible for people who want to develop stronger pelvic muscles.

Possible reasons for having weak pelvic muscles are:

Labor and Delivery

Pregnancy and delivery are leading causes of weakened pelvic muscles. Numerous modifications occur in the body of pregnant women to accommodate the developing fetus. Abdominal expansion, breast enlargement, plus general weight increase are all examples.

The hips, back and pelvis may experience extra strain as a result of all these alterations. It also puts strain on vagina, which may be harmful to the uterine arteries and nerves during labor and delivery. In addition, because of the weight of the baby pressing down on the bladder, you may find yourself unable to regulate your bladder needs throughout labor.

Surgery

Surgery, particularly abdominal and pelvic procedures, is another factor that might weaken pelvic muscles. This can happen after abdominal surgery, such a hysterectomy, a C-section, or the removal of the gallbladder. Most often, rectovaginal procedures may weaken the rectus and vaginal muscles that help keep your bladder, uterus and intestines healthy.

Injury, whether from a collision or physical activity, is another typical cause of weaker floor muscles. Because of this, pelvis may become skewed, and a reduction of elasticity in the tissues may make it hard to prevent organ prolapse. Bladder and uterus are organs most often damaged in this way.

Age

Weak floor muscles are more common as people age. This is because your muscles have weakened as a result of giving birth and natural aging. Bone loss, which may make moving around difficult; reduced levels of estrogen, which may lead to dryness in the vagina; constipation, urinary incontinence, and lack of control over the bladder (fecal incontinence); and other symptoms are all examples.

Conditions including arthritis, MS, Parkinson's disease, & spinal cord trauma have all been linked to weak floor muscles of pelvis.

Long Periods of Inactivity

Finally, not taking breaks from standing or sitting for an extended amount of time might lead to frail pelvic floor muscles. When you don't get up and move about, your muscles have to work harder to support your organs & to maintain you upright. If you have desk job that requires you to sit for long periods of time without standing up, this is very risky.

3.2 How Can I Tell If My Floor Muscles of Pelvis Are Weak?

These extend from where they join to pubic bone down into pelvic bones. Uterus & bladder both rely on them for support. They are out of sight and out of mind unless there is an issue. The following are symptoms that may indicate weak floor muscles of pelvis:

• Stress Incontinence

• Pelvic Pain

• Frequent Urination

If you identify with any of the following, it is possible that you have a weaker pelvic floor muscle. Just stop urinating in the middle, to be sure. If you can perform this without stopping, it's a good sign that muscles are sufficiently developed. Yet, weak muscles may be to blame if you have trouble stopping urine in its tracks or when you feel the need to urinate, regardless of whether nothing is coming out.

3.3 How is Nervous System impacted by Pilates?

The hormonal & chemical equilibrium of the human body is maintained by the autonomic nervous system, a subset of nervous system.

It's very perceptive to the little details of our lives. The body's parasympathetic & sympathetic reactions alternate throughout day. Only when we're paying very careful attention or when our neurological systems are about to break, then we become conscious of this shift. In a restful parasympathetic state, we feel calm, collected, and capable of sleeping well. We've reached an optimal condition where we're healthy, happy, and prepared to pick up new skills and bounce back swiftly from setbacks. Since there are no external dangers to contend with, our brain chooses to devote its resources to repairing and developing our bodies during this period. Among them are the functions of sleep, rest & digestion, healing, & learning.

The sympathetic nervous system (NS) is activated in response to increased pressure or stress. Minor alterations occur in our bodies, like an increase in blood tension and blood pressure that causes us to breathe more quickly and shallowly.

Our NS is hopelessly out of touch with modern times

It sees feelings of anxiety and stress as a defensive mechanism. In response, our bodies prepare for action (fight/flight).

As our sympathetic condition deepens, the NS begins to sacrifice other functions in order to ensure our immediate survival. It maintains mental and physical preparedness. The only thing our brain can do is zero in on the possible danger or unpleasant circumstance in front. There is limited time for recuperative sleep, intellectual ability, or damage recovery.

The sympathetic & parasympathetic nervous systems should cooperate in harmony for optimal health. On the other hand, we are no longer survivalists. Our neurological systems may not fully comprehend the lifestyles we lead. It has no concept of the difficulties associated with meeting employment obligations.

It has no knowledge of medical procedures or drugs. It doesn't get how much pressure we're under to stifle our feelings. This may interfere with our NS's ability to maintain its natural equilibrium.

We all understand that fatigue and anxiety are constant companions, but what percentage of us & our customers also struggle with concerns like elevated blood pressure, trouble sleeping, gastrointestinal disorders, muscular tension, memory loss, difficulty concentrating, and chronic pain? Adding another stressful incident, such as a death or an automobile accident, to an already unbalanced neural system might cause us to stay in sympathetic pattern much beyond our tolerance level. It might drive us too far into a para-sympathetic condition, also beyond our comfort zone. We understand that this is a depressive episode.

To suggest that a lot of us are now experiencing an unbalanced NS would be an understatement.

It's important to think about how this could be influencing our customers throughout their time with us. It's crucial that we're able to accurately assess our customers' emotional states upon their arrival.

Are they overburdened and fatigued, and are they speaking quickly and loudly as they hurry in?

Do they say they can't sleep or that they have stomach aches?

These behaviors are indicative of someone who is presently mired in sympathetic state. It's possible that if they start their workout in that state, they won't be able to relax into it and move freely throughout it. Their immune system is still on the lookout for danger. We don't want it since it will hinder their recovery, the development of new motor skills, and the acquisition of new patterns of motion.

Pilates and breathing techniques may be used to help reset the nervous system.

Relaxing the body & lowering one's stress levels are both necessary steps toward restoring equilibrium when nervous system disturbance is present. We like to place a lot of emphasis on two particular tactics for making that happen: breathing properly and doing Pilates. Even while they are not the only ways to self-regulate, they may be quite helpful on the road to recovery and getting back to a healthy state.

The encouraging news is that both of these factors, too, go in harmony hand with one another.

Both of these may help assist in the regulation of the nervous system in the following ways.

Breath

Put an immediate halt to what you're doing and focus on your breath. Focus your attention on the rhythm of the breath coming in and out.

• Do you breathe through your nostrils or through your mouth?

• Are you inhaling into the chest, the abdomen, or both at the same time?

Your present pattern of breathing can have an effect on both your general health and the way you are feeling right now. The details that one provides to the other are mutually beneficial for your neurological system & your respiratory system, which are good pals. Paying attention to the way you breathe might assist you in shifting into the appropriate mental state.

Both the manner in which we breathe & the condition of our minds are intricately tied to the neurological system. If you utilize the breath to relax your body & bring your attention to the here and now, you may change the mode of the nervous system from one of "flight/flight"(sympathetic activation) to one of "digestion and rest" (parasympathetic activation).

Breath work has the potential to slow down the amygdala, which sends the brain the signal that anxiety and fear are not needed at this time. In point of fact, research from 2016 indicates that practicing deep breathing might lower the amygdala's sensitivity to emotional cues. When practiced daily, this leads to a general state of relaxation throughout the body, which in turn helps regain control.

Movement, especially Pilates, may be an effective technique for soothing the nervous system. Even a brief bout of exercise may help your body produce "feel-good" chemicals, which are neurotransmitters like dopamine & serotonin. These neurotransmitters serve a role in modulating mood, boosting attention, and assisting the brain in operating more efficiently as a whole.

Because it emphasizes awareness of the present moment and controlled breathing, Pilates has been shown to lower levels of hormones associated with stress, like cortisol. This, in turn, may help us become less anxious and more at ease in our daily lives. Additionally, when we exercise our bodies, we boost blood flow, which helps to provide oxygen to brain, allowing us to process information more clearly (so long, brain fog!) and perform more effectively.

Pilates is among the greatest methods to connect the body and mind in order to not only improve strength, increase mobility, and lessen pain and discomfort but additionally to support healthy neurological system. Pilates is among the finest ways to promote an optimal nervous system.

3.4 How practicing Pilates may assist the body's reaction to stress.

MOVEMENT. The release of endorphins that make you feel good may occur as quickly as 10 minutes after engaging in exercise, and most of us are familiar with post-workout peaks that can be induced by exercise. Pilates also offers this benefit, but since the majority of the exercises are done at a somewhat slower tempo, include breathing control and mindfulness, and are accompanied by feel-good stretches & movements, we may often have an even stronger reaction to our training.

BREATHING. Pilates instructs students in a certain breathing rhythm. This is due to two very important factors. To begin, the physical activation of core muscles is more effective when it is performed on an exhale; as a result, you get more control over your muscles. Furthermore, when you move in time with your breath, you are able to produce a certain pace with the movement. This keeps you from working through the workouts too quickly. Lowering the pace at which you breathe not only serves to control the parasympathetic system, which is the portion of your neural system responsible for relaxing, but it also has the potential to lower your blood pressure, heart rate and overall sensation of anxiousness. You may check out some of my other suggestions for relaxing right here.

MINDFULNESS. Pilates is a kind of exercise that helps you strengthen the mind-body connection. This involves coordinating your movements, breath, and thoughts in such a way that both your body and mind are working together in unison. The nervous system may be helped to self-regulate and become more peaceful when you pay more attention and become more conscious. The actual performance of the exercises not only activates the mind-body link but also heightens your awareness of the interior workings of your body, which in turn activates autonomic system. This improves the activity of the vagus nerve, which originates in the brain and whose main task is to facilitate relaxation and reduce stress. Eighty percent of the job of the vagus nerve is to transmit messages from the body to the brain. That is a significant number of signals that are sent to our bodies whenever we engage in physical exercise.

ROUTINE. A consistent Pilates practice fosters routine. The process of doing your exercises on a regular basis, as well as the routine that you follow throughout your practice, consists of the sequence of prescribed exercises designed to address your upper body, core, lower body, & mobility/stretches. Brain is able to relax as a result of a regular pattern because this "safe" part of routine is something your body grows used to, which eliminates uncertainty and allows body to settle into a familiar procedure.

Chapter 4: Pilates and Chronic Conditions

The outcomes of Pilates as program for rehabilitation are employed for the management of chronic pain in low back, and the outcomes of Pilates might be matched to the outcomes of exercise programs. According to the findings of Cochrane Review, quality of evidence that supports the usefulness of Pilates as treatment for pain & impairment in instances of pain in low back is moderate to great. However, current research indicates that Pilates workout regimen for three to nine weeks, involving 1–2 practices per week that consist of core & strength exercises/mind–body workouts, has proven to be most beneficial way for dealing with disability and pain arising from chronic LBP.

4.1 Research on Pilates' Usefulness in Pain of Low Back

This program includes practices that focus on movements that target the core & strengthen the body. The vast majority of Pilates programs for low back pain focus on strengthening or engaging the core muscular group, sometimes known as "power house." Isometric contraction of deep muscles of abdomen, floor muscles of pelvis, gluteus maximus, & multifidus muscles is primary component of this exercise. The exercises included a 5-minute warm-up consisting of breathing & mobility exercises, followed by 50 minutes of Pilates exercises consisting of strengthening and stretching techniques for the trunk muscles as well as the lower & upper limbs, plus finally, a 5-minute cool-down consisting of relaxation activities including ball massage. Concentric plus eccentric contractions of the spine, trunk, upper & lower limb, and abdominal muscles were employed in the exercises. Movement was conducted in all planes of motion. The duration of the break between workouts was two minutes, and the number of repetitions ranged from eight to twelve. Based on Borg scale, these numbers corresponded to around sixty to seventy percent of one maximal repetition. The activities were carried out at three different difficulty stages: basic, intermediate, & advanced. The fundamental exercises were modified so that they were appropriate for each individual patient by either increasing or decreasing the amount of resistance (for example, roll-up activity that is carried out on Cadillac using tower bar may be carried out with spring in high position to render movement easier, and in low position to render movement additionally difficult).

There has been enough research done on Pilates exercises to determine whether or not they are beneficial in treating patients who suffer from chronic pain of low back. A study was conducted using three different questions, and it was given to thirty Australian physical therapy professionals who have expertise with Pilates exercises. Participants were in agreement that those that exhibit poor awareness of their bodies and dysfunctional patterns of movement could reap advantages from Pilates workouts. Furthermore, participants were in agreement that Pilates training may increase functional capacity as well as movement confidence, posture, body awareness & movement control.

An additional randomized controlled trial was carried out with the purpose of determining the impact that Pilates has on the postural alignment of adult women. According to the findings, Pilates-based training improved a number of features of postural alignments, which were evaluated by measuring frontal alignment of shoulders and sagittal alignment of head & pelvis.

4.2 The Correlation between Pilates& Parkinson's Disease

Parkinson's disease ranks as the world's second most prevalent kind of neurological illness. In spite of the fact that Parkinson's disease is most often seen in persons in their later years, 15% of those who have the condition are really under the age of 50, and in very rare instances, they are even in their 20s!

Parkinson's disease is characterized by the death of the nerve cells in brain, which play a role in the creation of dopamine &, as a result, the regulation of motion. The exact etiology of Parkinson's disease is unknown at this time, but we are certain that it leads to the condition.

The symptoms that you may encounter might vary considerably from individual to individual; however, the most common symptoms are stiffness, tremors, & slowness of mobility. The most significant challenge that most individuals confront is dysfunction in their mobility caused by these signs, which gradually may reduce their level of independence.

Regrettably, we are aware that signs will get more severe with time. But some therapies, like Pilates, have been shown to assist in enhancing life quality and decrease the progression of symptoms related to Parkinson's disease.

There is just a little amount of information available at this time that examines the advantages of Pilates for those who have Parkinson's disease. Nevertheless, some study into the utilization of Pilates for persons who have Parkinson's disease has indicated that increases in strength of lower limbs as well as independent functioning will translate into gains in functional mobility, enabling them to engage in daily activities with more safety & efficiency.

Even more convincingly, the evidence shows that "its benefits on lower-body function appear to be superior to those of other conventional exercises."

People who have Parkinson's disease can benefit from Pilates in number of other ways as well, including: increasing flexibility; enhancing balance & coordination; strengthening the mind-muscle link; enhancing general fitness; reducing discomfort; providing increased mobility.

Pilates is a fantastically adaptable kind of exercise that can be addressed from a wide variety of perspectives based on the desired outcomes.

When you have Parkinson's disease, the effect that Pilates has on your neurological system is among the most essential benefit you can get from the exercise.

Pilates is not so much about the movements themselves as it is about the manner in which they are performed. Because of this, you will need to pay attention to the way you move, that, in and of itself, may assist in achieving greater control of your motions as the symptoms progress. This is because we deal with methods that alter neuromuscular control, which has an effect not only on strength but additionally on nervous system as well as how it regulates your motions.

Pilates has traditionally been thought of as a way to strengthen the abdominal region, sometimes known as "power house." However, a more contemporary perspective demonstrates that it also helps to build strength & effective stimulation of local & global stabilizers, not just around spine but also at every joint. This not only improves the alignment of your spine and pelvis as well as the posture overall, but it is additionally a significant contributor to the development of stronger control over the movement.

We are aware that among the most prominent signs of Parkinson's disease are stiffness & rigidity of motion. The fact that Pilates places such a high value on using one's whole range of movement is a big advantage as one's symptoms progress. This is not an exercise designed to teach you how to do splits; instead, it is designed to assist you in preserving as much flexibility and motion throughout the body as is humanly feasible. The technique of Pilates places a strong emphasis on breathing, which in turn offers a wonderful supplementary aid for the facilitation of relaxation.

People often who have Parkinson's disease have problems commencing the movement (this is sometimes referred to by the term "freezing"), which means that whatever activity you get patients to undertake, they may require additional support and physical direction in the form of signaling and displays to get going with movement. Then, after they start moving, you should keep them continuing with that activity until tiredness comes in (you want to prevent continuously shifting and altering the activity after few repetitions).

The patient may have apparent shaking or tremors of limbs/body while engaging in physical activity. The degree of Parkinson's disease will determine whether or not this occurs. This is an instinctive response, and it is not a reason to refrain from completing the exercise (provided that patient is not experiencing any discomfort or pain).

If a patient suffers from pain, they should only exercise within range they can handle, which might entail potentially reducing range of motion.

Adjust training periods according to when it's most beneficial to you and end sessions earlier when necessary. Individuals may have more energy at various times of day; therefore schedule workouts around this (for example, many individuals with Parkinson's condition report feeling tired later in day). If that's the situation, you should schedule your session for morning.)

Be mindful that your balance may probably be disturbed, and make sure that you are secure whole time; have something sturdy to grab onto to help maintain equilibrium.

Parkinson's disease patients often exhibit the following symptoms:

• Tight as well as stiff through thoracic spine, particularly if they exhibit stooped posture that leads to bending through thoracic spine (increased kyphosis); focusing on mild thoracic extension as well as rotation stretches may assist with this

• Tight through Psoas as well as hip muscles; concentrating on mild mobility of the hips can aid with this

• Tight through Latissimus Dorsi

• Tight through chest and Pecs due to protracted and rounded shoulders

As symptoms of the illness progress, falling may become an increasingly dangerous risk and a significant source of anxiety. Not only can improving your body awareness, balance, and control of motion help lessen the likelihood of falling, but it additionally assists in minimizing the negative effects that falling may have on your daily life. As a result of this, including it as an essential component of the plan ought to be a priority. Four studies that compared participants' balance scores prior to and following Pilates treatments revealed considerable improvements, demonstrating how beneficial this exercise may be.

Fundamentally speaking, doing Pilates will assist in enhancing your strength, balance, mobility, control of motion, and posture, which will ultimately have a significant and favorable impact on your overall quality of life.

And the greatest part regarding Pilates is the fact that it is an exercise that you can start doing from the very beginning of the onset of the symptoms, and you can continue doing it even as they get more severe. In order to acquire these abilities, getting started as soon as possible after receiving your diagnosis is ideal. Once you've acquired an understanding of the fundamentals, the concepts, and a plan that is tailored to your needs, you will find that doing it at home is a breeze.

It should come as no surprise that the optimum treatment plan differs from individual to individual, much like symptoms. If you do have Parkinson's disease, though, here are some crucial components of your Pilates routine that you should include:

• Strength: all over the body

• Mobility: for maintaining your range of movement

• Coordination: to allow the limbs to keep trying to work on their own

• Balance: to assist you in avoiding falls

• Goal establishment: so you understand what you desire to accomplish!

4.3 Pilates as treatment for arthritis

The Disease Control & Prevention Center of USA reports that one in every four persons in the country is affected by arthritis, which is defined as the stiffness of one or more joints. Osteoarthritis, often known as destruction of cartilage that lines a joint is among the most prevalent kind of arthritis. Imagine cartilage as sort of cushion for shocks in your body. When the cartilage between the bones is destroyed, the outcome is grinding sound. Because of this, those with arthritis experience excruciating pain and are limited in their range of motion. This, consequently, is the root cause of a domino effect of other problems, such as an inability to hold down a job or carry out routine tasks.

Advantages of Pilates for People with Arthritis

Physical exercise has been shown to be effective in reducing the pain associated with arthritis, which may seem paradoxical. The proverb "drive it or destroy it" is applicable in this situation. Similar to how motor oil coats engine of the automobile, motion assists in keeping the pain & tightness of joints at bay. We additionally understand that regular exercise enhances our standard of life by boosting self-confidence, elevating mood, and reducing the symptoms of depression. For individuals who suffer from arthritis, the Centers for Disease Control and Prevention suggests participating in weekly physical exercise for a minimum of 150 mins at moderate levels of difficulty. This figure could make you feel overwhelmed, but remember that it can be broken down into manageable chunks and spread out over the course of day or week.

It is essential to choose the appropriate kind of physical activity in order to avoid exacerbating the discomfort associated with your arthritis. Anything that is disturbing to joints should be avoided by those who have osteoarthritis, in addition to people who have other types of arthritis like rheumatoid arthritis. Rather, you should search for low-impact workouts that may help you preserve your range of movement in your joints while also working on stretching, improving your breathing, and elevating your heart rate.

Reasons Pilates is Fantastic Option for Those Who Suffer from Arthritis

Due to these factors, Pilates is an excellent option for persons who suffer from arthritis. Pilates places emphasis on stability in the core, which assists with balance, in addition to spinal flexibility, which helps you accomplish the tasks of everyday life, such as driving and reaching goods on elevated shelves. In addition, doing Pilates may help you keep or enhance range of movement in your joints, which is something that is quite beneficial if you suffer from arthritis.

Exercises like Footwork & Leg Circles on Pilates Reformer device or Leg Springs performed on Cadillac, for instance, develop the muscles that surround hip, knee, & ankle joints without causing any impact. In a same manner, muscles of shoulder girdle may be strengthened by doing arm spring sequence, as well as Push Through& Roll Back movements on Cadillac or Pilates Tower. These big and tiny muscles work together to provide support for joints and facilitate movement that is more effective.

Where to Begin When you're suffering from arthritis in your joints.

Before starting any kind of workout routine, you should always be sure to check in with your primary care physician first. Once you have received permission from your physician, the next best thing would be to locate a trained instructor in your region who has prior experience dealing with those who suffer from arthritis. If feasible, take some individual lessons. The teacher may provide pointers that are catered specifically to you & your physique. If you decide to go to group courses, semi-private appointments, or perhaps online fitness sessions, you will acquire the knowledge necessary to alter routines. Be patient with yourself as you are getting started. It is preferable to ease into something and maintain a steady pace rather than push yourself too hard and risk injury or exhaustion.

Alterations to Pilates Routines for Arthritis

If you are participating in a collaborative class, you should get there early in order to inform the teacher of any limitations, which are defined as activities or motions that your doctor has advised you to steer clear of or that cause you pain. It is possible that you may discover that you must tailor some workouts to the way your body works in order to get the most out of them. If you suffer from arthritis in the knees, for instance, you may need to steer clear of positions that require a deep bending of knee joint, such as resting on the heels while sitting in Child's Posture. You may stretch lower back by placing a rolled-up cloth behind the knees, or you may opt for another posture, such as standing or lying.

Warming up prior to exercise may assist ease mobility and reduce the likelihood of experiencing discomfort. This might be going for a stroll or even doing something as simple as having a warm bath or shower prior to session. Pay attention to your bodily cues. Do not ignore the throbbing in your chest. You should pause what you're doing, take a break, and either attempt a new exercise or an altered version of activity you were doing.

Do not be disheartened if you get sore after the initial few exercises since this is a common and expected reaction to beginning a new fitness routine. If, on the other hand, you do not begin to feel improved or if you begin to feel more discomfort, you should re-evaluate your activity and speak to your physician about selecting a kind of physical activity that is more suited to your needs.

4.4 Is Pilates Risk-Free?

In a word, absolutely, but only if you understand your limits!

Concerns about how secure you feel & whether or not you believe something is doable are quite prevalent for those who have Parkinson's disease.

Pilates poses a very minimal chance of injury when it is performed with the correct technique, and furthermore, the movements should be adapted to you, thereby rendering it suitable for anybody, regardless of their ability and stage of life.

For instance, if your primary fear is falling, we may modify each Pilates practice to help increase your trust in yourself to ensure you are able to move & grow powerful without feeling wobbly or in danger. This will allow you to take advantage of the benefits that Pilates offers. This might involve utilizing the assistance of equipment, maintaining your position on floor, or seeking support while doing balancing exercises. You also require no assistance to get on & off floor, which is a significant benefit if you are having trouble with movement in question.

You should see your physician before beginning any kind of physical activity and conduct some research to find out who you should visit and who seems like a good fit for you to collaborate with. Because of COVID, it is now possible to collaborate with someone who lives in another town or perhaps in another region of the globe than you do!

Pilates incorporates a wide variety of methods and systems, and it may be practiced in a variety of settings, ranging from big groups to individual instruction. The most important thing is to locate something & someone that's beneficial for you. It is also essential that the individual in issue have the necessary credentials; thus, you should not be scared to inquire about this.

4.5 The advantages of Pilates for those with ongoing medical conditions

The Reformer and the Mat Pilates is increasingly being acknowledged as a vital therapeutic practice that improves both qualities of life and health. Exercises function by improving the main muscle support system, which in turn offloads joints and leads to a decrease in discomfort in joints. This may lower pain for variety of medical disorders and thus can contribute to a decrease in overall pain.

The exercises have a minimal risk of injury, improve both flexibility and strength and are tailored to each individual condition.

Conditions related to health care

Multiple Sclerosis: enhance stability & strength of your core muscles to lower your chance of falling while improving your balance and mobility. Pilates may help alleviate pain and exhaustion, as well as improve cognitive function and performance, all of which contribute to a heightened awareness of one's physical posture. Increase the distance covered by walking. Improve one's life quality and general sense of well-being.

Heart issues: Pilates has been proven to promote heart health in individuals with cardiovascular diseases by improving their breathing & functional capacity, reducing both physical and mental stress, and considerably improving their metabolic function. This research was conducted on people who already had heart disease.

Fibromyalgia: Pilates places a focus on breathing methods to soothe muscles and avoid tension, which may be helpful for those who suffer from fibromyalgia. The process of oxygenating the blood and increasing circulation to all parts of the body is called breathing. People often who suffer from fibromyalgia have a tendency to detach from their bodies. The integration of one's mind and body is at the heart of the Pilates method. It aids in the prevention of hypermobility and lessens the feelings of exhaustion that are linked with fibromyalgia.

Pilates has been shown to be effective in bringing down elevated cholesterol levels. The Pilates routine demonstrated substantial rises in HDL-C blood concentration even with a rise in ratio of body fat, indicating that Pilates activity was beneficial for boosting lipid metabolism in blood, especially with increasing levels of HDL-C. HDL, or good cholesterol, assists in eliminating cholesterol from the arteries.

Diabetes: Pilates improves insulin's ability to act, which increases the likelihood of improved diabetes control and helps diabetics and those at risk for diabetes decrease their blood sugar levels.

4.6 Advice on Preventing Injuries for Senior Citizens

1. Be sure to follow the instructions

It is possible that the exercises the elderly person does need to have some modifications made to them in order to lessen the danger of strains & accidents. Altering movement in any way might, however, pose a risk to the participant's safety. When making modifications to the prescribed exercises for you, it is important to check in with your primary care physician first. This will allow you to determine which activities are appropriate for you and which modifications might raise the likelihood of harm occurring. You may safely exercise in the comfort and privacy of your own home with assistance of a trained caregiver.

2. Don't Overstep It

Although the schedule that you adopt ought to be demanding, it should not be too taxing on their mental capacity. If the person you care about puts too much pressure on themselves, they run the risk of injuring muscle or breaking a bone. You need to be aware of the limitations that the body can withstand and should make every effort to remain within those bounds.

3. Ensure that you are Outfitted Properly

Wearing workout clothing that is either too loose or too tight, as well as trousers that are too big, might increase the chance of injury. When moving, for instance, you may have muscular tension if the clothes you are wearing are overly constricting. If the footwear you are wearing is too big or too small, there is an increased risk that you may trip and either break bone or suffer a brain injury. It is important for you to have the right gear on whenever you go outside to exercise, whether you are at home working out or going on walks, runs, or bike rides around the neighborhood.

4. Get Warmed Up Properly

It is possible to lessen the likelihood of experiencing muscular pain by doing a pre-workout warmup that includes stretching. You will boost the core temperature and experience a rise in blood circulation to muscles while participating in warmup. It could be beneficial for your parent to have a period of time to relax once they have finished exercising.

5. Always Be Aware Of Your Environment

When engaging in physical activity, you should always keep a vigilant watch on what's going on in the immediate vicinity in order to maximize safety. It is not advisable for an elderly person who struggles with sight/hearing to engage in physical activity in the absence of a family member or another adult in good health. Your cognitive decline, problems with memory, poor eyesight, & hearing loss are all severe safety concerns that may be mitigated with the assistance of a caregiver. The caretaker can help you prevent bumping into items and falling. There are numerous different scenarios in which elderly people could need help at home. A finding of Alzheimer's disease may cause some people to need consistent mental stimulation, whilst a diagnosis of dementia may cause others to need just part-time support with exercise & basic housekeeping duties.

6. Be sure to stay hydrated.

Seniors run the risk of falling victim to dehydration at any point in time, particularly when they are physically active. If you do not consume sufficient amounts of water along with other healthful fluids, you may suffer from muscular cramps, migraines, and a general feeling of weakness. When engaging in physical activity, the person you care about should drink lots of fluids to avoid becoming lightheaded and experiencing a drop in blood pressure. Because the care requirements of each elderly person are unique, it is not necessary for all of them to get the same kind of in-home assistance.

4.7 Modifications and Safety Measures to Take

For seniors who are suffering from osteoporosis

Pilates is beneficial for older adults with osteoporosis; however participating in a regular Mat Pilates session is not a good idea for these individuals. If you have osteoporosis, you should avoid using Roll Up, Jack Knife, Roll Over, Spine Twist, & Saw activities from the Mat workout because they provide a risk of injury. Many other Mat exercises may be adapted for increased safety. You should avoid doing any activities that require rolling on the back, bending forward, or rotating at spine because of the risk of injury. Taking an exercise class or having an individual lesson with Pilates instructor who is knowledgeable about the things that should and should not be done while doing Pilates exercises for osteoporosis is a fantastic idea in general.

Senior Citizens Who Have a Restricted Range of Movement

Among the nicest things regarding Pilates is the fact that it can adapt to the body no matter what state it's in right now. In the event that you have a restricted range of movement, you might adjust your practice such that it better accommodates your limitations. Do not attempt to force a move in any direction. We suggest that you move more carefully and slowly, relying on your breath as a source of support. Stay inside your range of movement while you train since the finest work can be accomplished.

Seniors that suffer from Arthritis

Pilates is beneficial for senior people who struggle with joint pain due to arthritis or another condition. However, development may be sluggish, and it is essential to avoid or alter workouts that exhaust the joints or strain them in any way. Exercises such as Roll Over, Spine Twist, Jack Knife, & Rolling Like Ball are examples of those that should be avoided. Keep in mind that mindfulness and attention are two of the most essential elements of Pilates method. Pay particular attention to the way you move as well as how you feel prior to beginning, during, and following the Pilates exercises. Do not engage in any activity that causes your joints or spine to feel uncomfortable. Working with a certified Pilates instructor who has completed training in Pilates treating arthritis & joint difficulties will increase the likelihood that you will get the results you want.

To Prevent Injury

It's common to find that senior Pilates pupils are far better at listening to and reacting to the cues their bodies give them than younger individuals. This is due to the fact that younger individuals often choose to "push through" stuff before they're actually ready, which causes them to disregard messages/pain signals that our bodies provide us. When doing Pilates, safety should at all times be your first priority. A qualified instructor will tell you to take it easy, instruct you to proceed within a more limited range of movement, and provide you with other ways to do the exercise. In order to improve your Pilates practice, it is a good idea to seek assistance and book a few one-on-one sessions alongside a qualified instructor. If a certain workout is causing you pain, you should stop performing it right away. As Pilates student, one of the most important things you can do is learn to listen to the body.

Book Two

Workout and Stretching

Chapter 1: Stretching Before Pilates

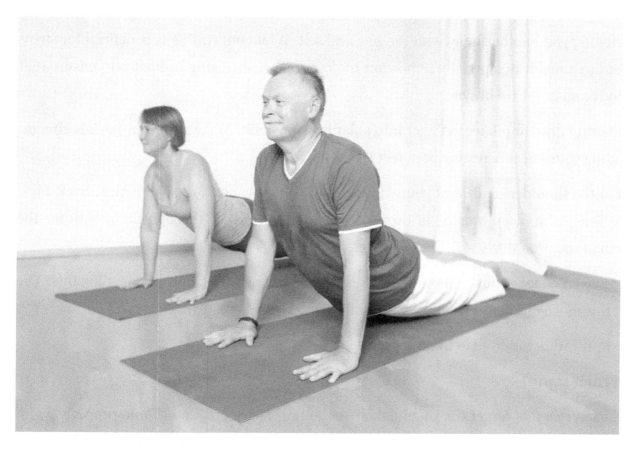

Is stretching important before Pilates?

To get maximum benefit out of a Pilates session, you need to warm up first. If you don't take the time to warm up beforehand, your body will have to rush through the procedure when it's not ready.

1.1 How About Some Pre-Pilates Stretches?

Extensive stretching is not recommended before Pilates lessons. In most cases, strenuous physical activity, such as yoga or Pilates equipment usage, is unnecessary and even counterproductive.

However, there are several stretches & mat exercises that have proven effective for Pilates that we recommend before lessons. You shouldn't feel pressured to do all of these motions before each Pilates session.

Instead, create a plan that will enable you to properly warm up the whole body before beginning Pilates. Start out with these 6 stretches:

Pilates Imprinting

Pilates imprint is very basic prone activity that aids in waking each and every muscle in body and bringing you into harmony with the physical self. While imprinting is beneficial for stress relief at any time, it is especially important to do so before engaging in Pilates to ensure that your body and mind are in sync.

• Whether on floor or pilates mat, get into a flat back position. Make sure your back is straight by bending your knees & resting both feet level on floor.

• Start at the shoulders and work your way down to your jaw, neck, ribs, abdomen, back, hips, & legs. Take calm, deep breaths in through the nose and exhale through the mouth for the duration of the procedure.

• Feel the spine elongating, loosening, and extending out against floor in your thoughts. The title of this move originates from the vertebral impressions it creates.

• Keep imprinting for three to five breaths.

Arm reach & pull

Pilates exercises that target the shoulders are essential. Therefore, you should properly warm up the arms & shoulders prior to using Pilates apparatus or doing the sorts of strenuous exercises often seen in Pilates sessions.

• Position your feet on floor almost shoulder-width distant, and stand erect. Raise the arms in straight line next to the body, wrists erect, but fingers relaxed.

• Reach forward & open the shoulder blades as you take a deep breath in.

• When you exhale, bring your shoulders back to a neutral posture while keeping the arms extended.

• Take a deep breath in as you draw the arms back & squeeze the blades of your shoulder together.

• Relax your shoulders & lower your arms as you let out a deep breath.

Pelvic Thrust

This simple thrusting exercise, often known as pelvic curl, gently engages the abdominal & leg muscles while lifting pelvis off floor. This move is more strenuous than the others on our list of recommended warm-ups, so you may want to save it for the conclusion of your stretching routine.

• Start with Sequential Breathing

• As you let your breath out, contract your abs to lower the pelvis toward the ground.

• Next, press the feet down & lift your tailbone while taking a deep breath in. Hips first, then raise lower back, then upper back.

• Maintain a vertical line from the pelvis to the shoulder blades, and lower the pelvis down toward the ground while you exhale.

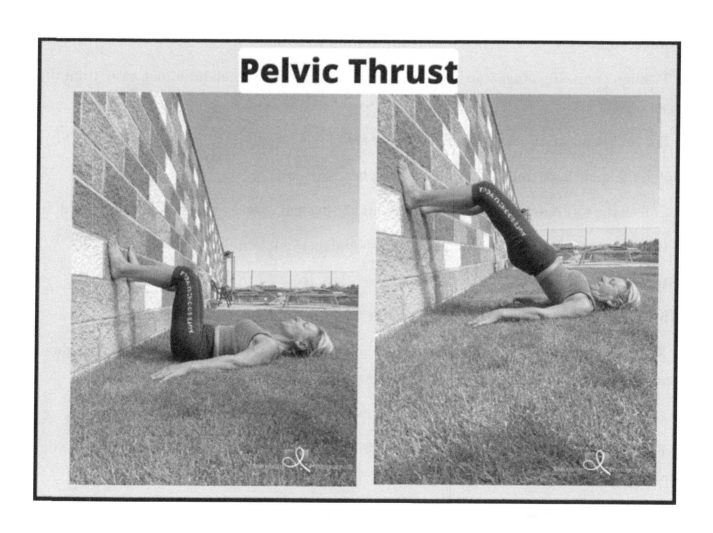

Swan prep

This is a variation on the standard Superman stretch in which the practitioner lifts his or her head off floor but keeps his or her feet on ground. If you choose, you may go to a complete Superman pose, which involves the same motions but different hand and foot positions as you elevate your head.

• Get on your stomach and lay there. Put the hand on floor close to the body while bending your elbows.

• Lift the belly off the floor by tightening your abs. Extend the back as you take a deep breath in.

• To bring your belly back to the mat, exhale and relax your spine in a series of movements.

Downward Pilates wall rolls

This Pilates warm-up doesn't need anything special—just a regular wall in the home. Put your bare feet on floor or mat, and become ready to work your abs.

• Position yourself so that your back is against wall and feet are about a foot away from the floor.

• Lift your hands over head and contract your abs.

• Roll the spine back from wall while nodding head forward.

• Roll all the way down while maintaining your abs pushed in and your butt against the wall.

• Inching your way back up to standing, you should feel your vertebras touching the wall.

Stretch of spine

Think of your body as tight "C" shape. That's the gist of the Pilates back stretch.

• Maintain a straight spine when you sit on floor with the butt planted. Split your legs about shoulder-wide apart after stretching them forward.

• Raise arms up & forward, palms pointing down, while you inhale.

• Exhale and lean forward from the hips, keeping the legs straight. Maintain a C-curve in your spine.

• To return to the beginning posture, elevate your torso using adequate spinal articulation.

Stretch of Spine

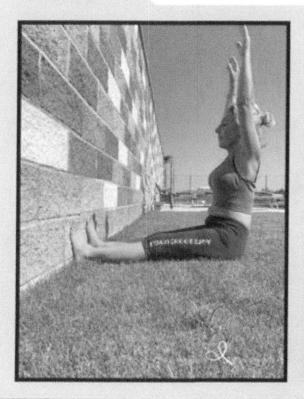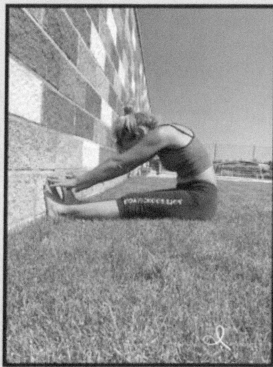

1.2 Full-Body Pilates Wall Exercise Example

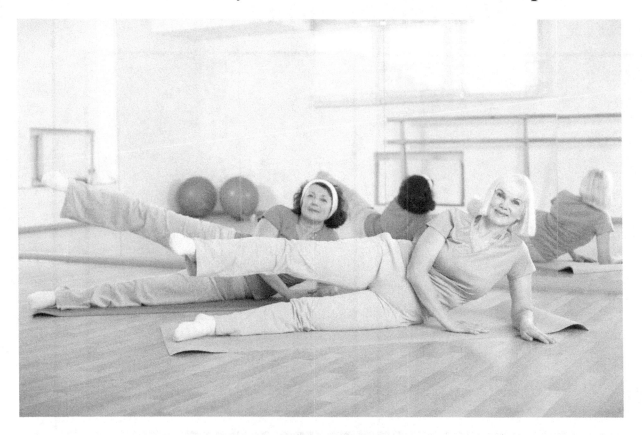

When starting out, it is advised that you do wall pilates no less than twice per week; however, many people find that performing the exercises three times per week tends to be even more helpful. Pilates may be done on a regular basis if recovery is given the proper amount of attention. Recovery occurs as the muscles grow and mend themselves.

It may take some time before you see results and improvements, so try to be patient. It's possible that the workouts that are the most challenging for you are also the most helpful.

Having a schedule will make it easier for you to keep track of and evaluate your advancement, & as you grow, you'll be able to modify your program & add to it as necessary.

Required equipment: Mat (optional) and Wall.

Warm-Up:

Assisted Roll down

1. Face a wall while standing tall. While keeping your back flat against wall, step away six inches.

2. Engage core. Maintain shoulder in relaxed position away from the ears.

3. Breathe in as you move spine down wall. As you drop, you should feel the back muscles elongating.

4. As you get to bottom of roll, breathe out. Keep the arms at your sides parallelly.

5. Retain for a few breaths. While you roll up back to starting position, take a breath in.

6. Repeat roll down five more times.

Hip opener (Standing)

1. Place 1 hand on wall to provide support as you begin to stand close to it.

2. Lift your outer leg till your thigh is level to the ground. Keep the pelvis square to front & level.

3. Use your inner hand as support by placing it on your lifted thigh.

4. As you breathe out, open the leg to side & gently push your lifted leg into hand.

5. Retain for a few breaths. As you let go of your leg and return it to beginning position, inhale.

6. Proceed to other side and repeat.

Leg swing (Side)

1. Place 1 o 2 hand on wall to provide support as you begin to stand close to it.

2. Lift your outer leg till the thigh is level to the ground. Keep the pelvis square to front & level.

3. Swing the leg upward outward to side as possible while maintaining a level pelvis.

4. Switch directions and return the leg to beginning position.

5. Continue on other side.

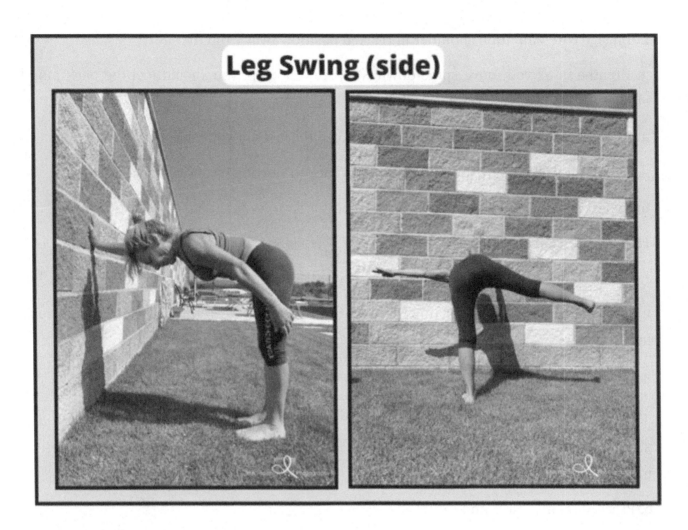

Leg Swing (side)

Calf stretch (Active)

1. Place your hands at the level of your shoulders against wall as you stand next to it.

2. Step back around two feet with the left leg, keeping your heel level on the ground.

3. While maintaining an erect left leg, bend the other knee & lean against wall until the left calf is stretched.

4. Retain for a few breaths. Continue on the opposite side after letting go.

Primary Set:

Supported Half Lunge

1. Place 1 hand on wall to provide support as you begin to stand close to it.

2. Place your left hand flat on wall and step with left leg backward approximately two feet.

3. While keeping the heel on the ground, bend the right knee and slant your body forward until the left hamstring starts to stretch.

4. Retain for a few breaths. Repeat on opposite side after letting go.

Knee Raise (Standing)

1: Begin by standing close to wall and placing one hand there for support.

2. Squeeze your stomach in and bring the right knee up to your chest.

3. Drive the lower back against wall while you lift your knee.

4. Retain for a few breaths. Repeat on opposite side after letting go.

Arm Raise (Wall DB)

1. Stand against wall, hold small dumbbells in both hands and bend your elbows to 90 degrees.

2. Hold your core firmly in place as you gently lift the arms until they're level to floor.

3. After a few moments of holding, return the arms to their initial position.

Arm Circles (Walls DB)

1. With the elbows bent at an angle of 90 degrees and a small dumbbell in both hands, stand against wall.

2. Hold your core firmly in place as you gently lift the arms until they're level to floor.

3. After that, do brief circular motions in air for thirty seconds.

4. Reverse the circles' direction and go on for an additional 30 seconds.

Chest opener

1. Place your feet approximately two feet from wall and stand with the back to the wall.

2. At the level of your shoulders, rest palms flat on the wall.

3. Brace the core and drive your chest toward the wall while sliding the hands up wall until the arms are completely stretched above.

4. Hold for one or two breaths before releasing to return to the beginning position.

Wall sits

1. Place your feet approximately two feet from wall and stand with the back to the wall.

2. Slide down wall gradually until the thighs are level to the ground.

3. Maintain this posture for as much time as you can, but at least 30 seconds.

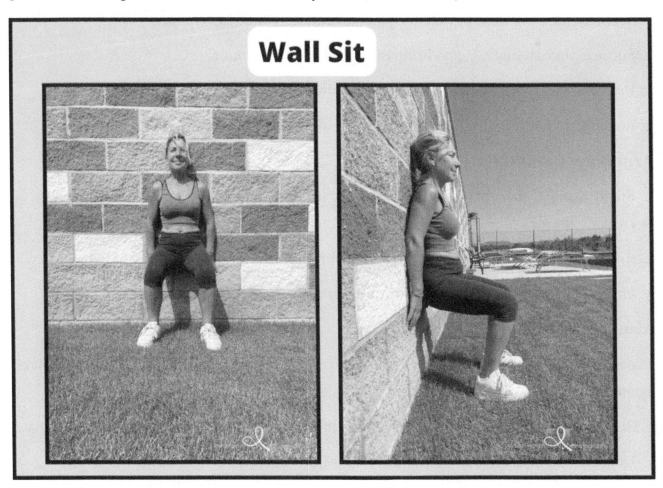

Cool Down

Toe Tap (Seated Opposite)

1. Begin by sitting down on floor with the legs straight in front and the back against wall.

2. Spread the legs out to around hip-width distance.

3. Engage your core muscles and push into wall with the lower back.

4. Extend the left hand and tap the right toe from this position.

5. Hold for 45 sec. on one side and repeat with the other side.

Spine Twist (seated)

1. Begin by sitting down on floor with the legs straight in front and the back against wall.

2. Spread the legs apart to around hip-width distance.

3. Brace the core.

4. Next, turn your body to right while extending the left hand to touch the floor just outside of right leg.

5. Turn the other way and extend the right hand to outside of the left leg and touch ground.

6. Hold for 45 seconds and repeat in opposite direction.

Butterfly Stretch

1. Position yourself in a sitting position on ground with the back against wall and the legs folded in front, with soles of feet touching.

2. Press the low back toward the wall while letting your knees hang wide to sides.

3. Next, arch the back out from wall while raising your arms above.

4. Hold for one or two breaths before releasing to return to the beginning position.

Forward fold (Seated)

1. Position yourself in a sitting position on ground with the back against wall and the legs folded in front, with the soles of your feet touching.

2. Press the low back against the wall while letting your knees hang wide to sides.

3. Next, bend forward from hips while letting the head & shoulders hang slackly. Raise the arms up while you do this.

4. Hold for one or two breaths before releasing to return to the beginning position.

Forward Fold (Seated)

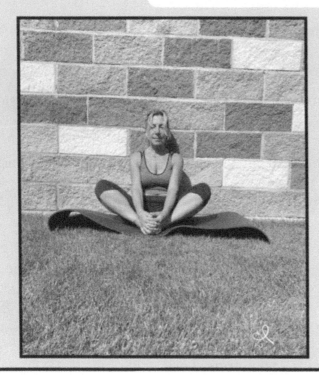 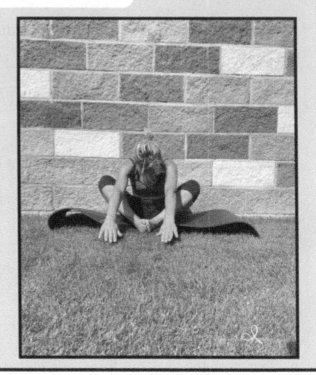

Chapter 2: Pilates Exercises

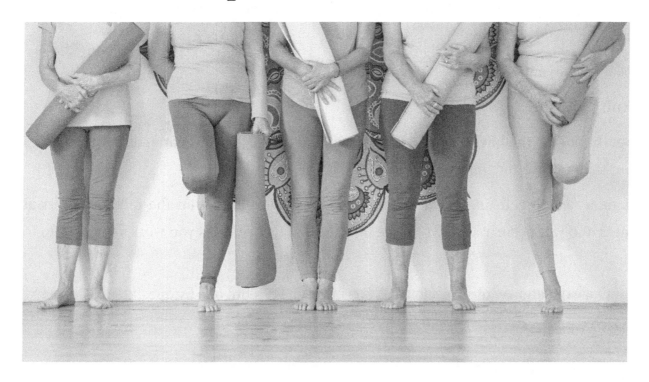

2.1 Easy And Fun To Do Exercise

Spinal Twist

1. Go into spinal twist posture, but keep your legs hanging to right side.

2. Inhale. When you let out your breath out, reach your left hand above the head and clasp it with the other hand. The sensation is similar to that of clam closing its shell.

3. The left shoulder will rise sharply off the ground. Come back to square one with an inhale.

4. Repeat 4 times, then switch sides and do it again.

Hip Looseners

Pilates movements like leg pull-downs, leg circles & kicks all rely on the participant having a high degree of hip mobility. Use hip releases & hip rolls to get your hips loose.

Hip Release

1. Get on the back with the knees bent & your feet flat on the floor. Take a deep breath in while you drop right knee to side outwards, creating the shape of butterfly wing.

2. Breathe out and extend right leg flat against the floor. Keep leg on the mat as you inhale and point the toes upward. While releasing your breath, bring your right knee back until your foot is flat on floor.

3. Repeat 4 times and switch sides to repeat the same sequence.

Hip Roll

1. Lie on back with the knees bent & your feet placed hip-distance separated. Fill your lungs with air, then release and imprint.

2. Taking a deep breath in, try rolling the spine up from floor from the tailbone. Start at shoulders and work your way down to the hips, forming a bridge as you work your way up to the toes.

3. let out an exhalation while consciously lowering each vertebra one by one.

4. Repeat 5 times.

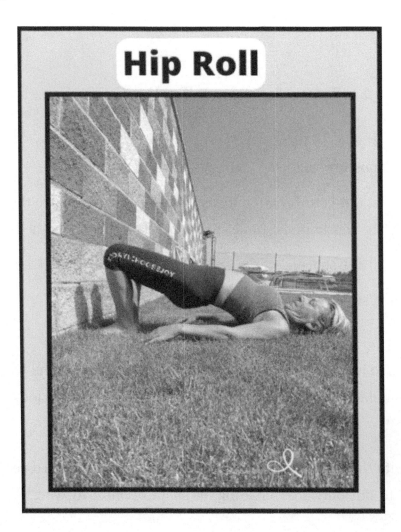

Flexing and extending the back

To make forward & backward bending of the spine easier, you should roll onto your stomach. If your body is feeling tight, try some of these active stretches. While cobra stretch enlivens lumbar spine and stretches fronts of shoulders and chest, cat stretch widens the back.

Cat stretch

1. Go down on all fours. Relax your back and breathe in.

2. While exhaling, draw belly button down toward spine & spine up into the ceiling, creating dramatic arch.

3. Take a deep breath in and keep your chin tucked and the tailbone rounded.

4. Exhale and form the natural position of back.

5. Repeat 5 times.

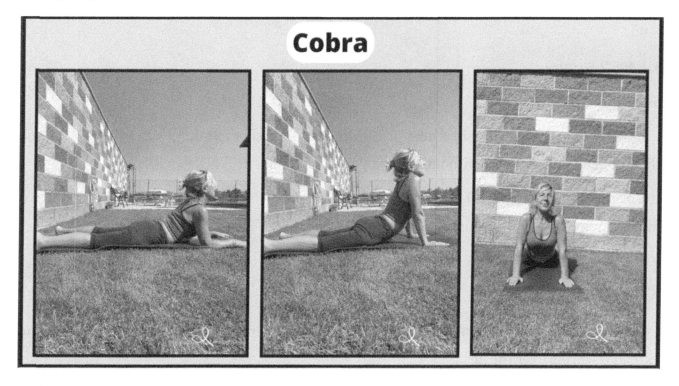

Cobra

1. Lie face down on a yoga mat. Hands should be beneath shoulders, elbows should be pointing upwards, & arms should be held tight to the body.

2. Inhale, then lift your head & chest off floor.

3. Exhale & sit back down. Keep the hands light & your back long as you lift.

4. Repeat 5 times.

Warming up the Upper Body

To conclude the warm-up, relax the muscles of upper body. While core is primary emphasis of Pilates, poor form may be compromised by tension in neck, shoulders, and arms. Spend a few more minutes to completely relax these muscles.

Head Nod

1. Lie on back with knees bent, with feet placed hip-distance separated. Keep the back in neutral position without imprinting or arching. Lay arms down on mat so they're next to your hips.

2. Take a deep breath in and stretch the back of the neck by reaching the head back; this will cause the chin to tuck ever-so-slightly. Release your breath and go back to where you were before. The movement is hardly perceptible, but it alerts you to muscles at the base of your skull.

3. Repeat 5 times.

Shoulder Shrug

1. Lie on back with knees bent & feet placed hip-distance separated. As you inhale, bring the shoulders up near the ears without moving your head or back.

2. Let out a deep breath & let them go. Do not round the shoulders. Only the up and down movements should be considered.

3. Repeat 5 times.

Arm Circle

1. Lie on back with knees bent & feet placed hip-distance separated. Take a deep breath in and extend the arms over the head.

2. Take a deep breath out, and move them to rest along the hips.

3. Repeat 3-5 times, then turn around and go in the other way, first looping out to sides and then above.

Arm Circle

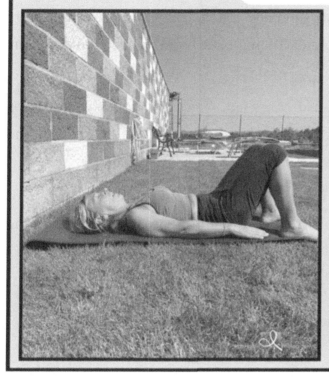 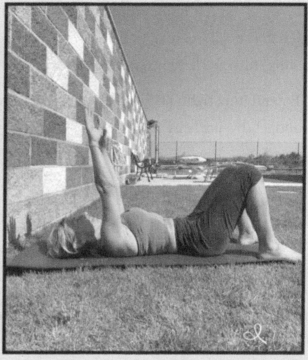

Roll into bridge upwards

1. Sit down with your face towards wall, and the knees bent. As you roll over onto the back, position your feet so that they are flat on wall and approximately hip-width separated. Your knees need to be bent around ninety degrees.

2. Raise the arms to the level of your chest while keeping your elbows straight. As you rise up to sitting posture, 1 vertebra at once, engage the muscles of your core, bring the chin to the chest, and lift your arms.

3. Roll backward until you reach the ground, 1 vertebra at once, and lay the arms on ground at the sides while you do so.

4. Bring the pubic bone closer to your navel as you push your feet toward the wall and elevate the hips into complete bridge posture.

5. Once again, bring the pubic bone into your navel as you drop your back & hips to floor 1 vertebra at once.

6. Perform the same steps ten times in a row.

Kneeling to Side with Leg Lift

1. Come into high-kneeling stance with the left side towards the wall. Bring the left side down and place your left hand on mat just under your shoulder. Extend the right leg of your body and put the sole of the right foot on the ground. To improve both your comfort & your stability, turn the left knee outward.

2. Extend the right arm so that it is positioned overhead. You may target your triceps &obliques by pressing against the wall with your right hand using either the palm or the fingers.

3. Point right toes & elevate the right leg until it is about hip level. Then, bring the right foot down until the toes are suspended an inch or two above ground. Repeat while maintaining proper leg level with torso.

4. Perform 10 repetitions on each side.

Bridge with a Single Leg, including Abduction

1. Sit down with face against the wall, and the knees bent. As you roll back onto the spine, position your feet so that they are flat on wall and approximately hip-width separated. Your knees need to be bent around ninety degrees. Put your arms down by the sides and rest them on ground.

2. While keeping your left foot pressed toward the wall, extend the right knee and point the toes in a straight upward direction toward ceiling.

3. Bring the pubic bone closer to your navel as you elevate the hips into complete bridge posture by pressing left foot toward wall. Use the muscles in your core to maintain the pelvis level.

4. Starting in bridge position, abduct (move out to side) the right leg by dragging it out from the center of your body. Don't go any farther than you are able to when feeling like your right hip is starting to drop.

5. Bring your right thigh back toward the center. While you lower the back & hips to floor 1 vertebra at once, be sure to tuck the pubic bone into your navel.

6. Perform for ten repetitions, and then switch sides. Repeat on the other side.

Side Plank, Including Rotation

1. Face the wall with the back, place the left palm beneath your left shoulder, move your feet apart, raise your hips, and stretch the right hand toward ceiling.

2. Bring the right arm down & beneath your torso, then stretch your hand out to contact the wall. Allow the hips to rise ever-so-slightly while you twist your body.

3. Come into a side plank position and extend right arm such that the fingers on the right hand are pointing up toward ceiling.

4. Perform 10 repetitions in a row, and then change sides. Repeat on the other side.

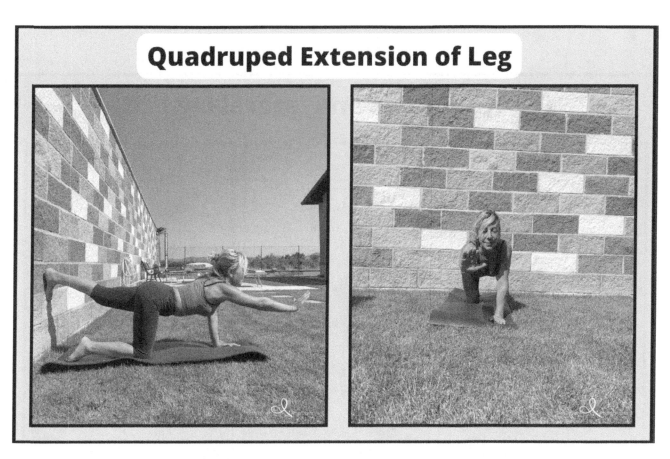

Quadruped Extension of Leg

1. Position yourself so that you are facing wall and go down on the hands and knees. Place the wrists under the shoulders and the knees under the hips. Maintain flat back while activating your core to improve your performance.

2. Raise the right arm until it is level with your shoulder, then push the palm of your right hand on the wall while simultaneously bringing your shoulder blade (right) down & back. Be sure that you're not too near to wall where you cannot fully extend the elbow while ensuring you are also not too far back that you cannot fully push against the wall.

3. Extend the left leg behind and point the left toes. Raise the left leg such that it is at or above hip height, but be sure to maintain the pelvis level while you do so. Reduce the distance between your toes and the floor to a few inches by lowering the leg. Repeat.

4. To make this exercise more difficult, curl the toes of your right foot under and do leg raises from hovering position.

5. Complete 10 repetitions on each side.

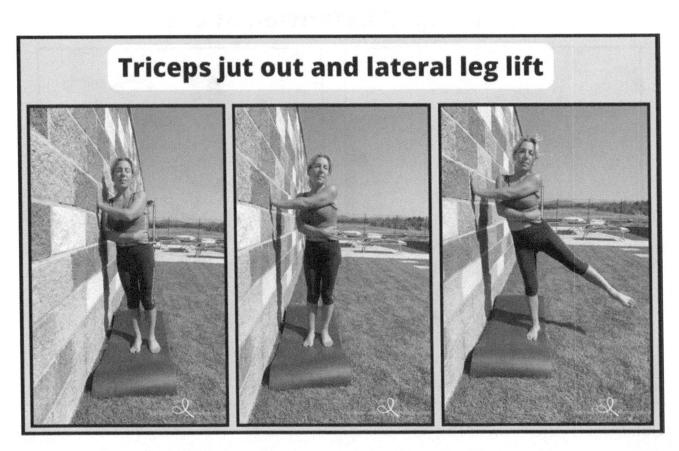

Triceps jut out and lateral leg lift

Triceps jut out and lateral leg lift

1. Stand with both feet together and left side of body toward the wall. Your palm should be on wall as you cross the right arm past your chest. Ensure that you are both near enough to wall in order to push against it and sufficiently far away in order to straighten the elbow. Wrap arm around midsection or move across chest.

2. Move your feet slightly away from wall so that you are leaning against it. (The exercise is harder the further apart the feet are from wall.)

3. Extend the elbow completely and bend the right arm to position your body close to wall. Next, push back from wall using your triceps.

4. Lift the right leg to around knee height while keeping the right knee straightened and foot flexed without letting the foot touch the ground, lower leg.

5. Follow the same pattern 10 times before switching sides. Repeat on the other side.

Wall roll down

The simplest movement you may do during the wall Pilates session is a roll-down. It is a straightforward standing workout that stretches back plus hamstrings and works the abs as well. You may begin your workout with a roll-down as way to warm up.

To do wall roll-down

• stand upright with the back against wall. Then, while maintaining your back pushed against wall, step your feet out at least 5 inches.

• Now, tighten your abdominal muscles as you gently roll the back down wall, making sure the arms are level to the sides.

• Repeat exercise after slowly rolling back to the beginning position.

Semi-lunge with support

The quadriceps, glutes and hamstrings are just a few of the significant muscles of the lower body that are worked during this specific wall Pilates activity. It strengthens knees and enhances hip stability.

• Stand close to wall with a hand on wall for stability in order to do aided semi-lunge.

• At this point, take one step back with the right leg and press the palm of your right hand on the wall. When you notice stretch in the right hamstring, slightly bend the left knee while keeping the heel down.

• Hold position before going back to the beginning. Before swapping sides, perform a few times.

Knee Crunch with Single-Leg

• Sit approximately a foot farther from wall and lie on the back. Your legs should be in tabletop posture as you place the feet level on wall.

• Extend the left leg diagonally so that your toes barely touch the wall. Brace your core by raising your arms above and pressing the lower back into ground. Your starting point is here.

• Lift shoulders off floor while drawing your left leg in toward the chest. To move arms adjacent to hips, draw them toward wall.

• Performing slow release, return to the beginning position. That is one rep.

• Perform 15 repetitions, then switch to right leg.

Calf Raise with Wall Bridge

• Lie on the back after positioning yourself approximately a foot back from wall. To position your legs on tabletop, place the feet level on wall. Your starting point is here.

• To activate your glutes and hamstrings and raise hips off floor, drive your feet firmly toward wall. (Ensure that back is not arched.) Lift the heels from wall to stabilize on the toes, then do calf raise once your body is in straight line from the knees to shoulders.

• To return to the beginning position, do the exercise in reverse by lowering the heels to wall first, followed by the hips to floor. That is one rep.

• Perform 15 repetitions.

Reach Backs

• Place your feet approximately a mat width separated in high plank posture, with balls of feet pushing against the wall. The body should make straight line from heels to shoulders, with your shoulders exactly above your wrists. Your starting point is here.

• Extend the hand (right) back to touch the ankle, left foot or shin while you lift the hips up & back into the Downward Dog position.

• Next, bring the hand (right) back to floor to get back into plank position and go back to beginning position. This is one rep.

• Continue by extending left hand in the direction of right ankle next.

• Perform ten repetitions per side.

Marching Bridge

• Lie on the back and position yourself approximately a foot farther from wall. To ensure that the legs lie on tabletop, place the feet level on wall. To raise hips off ground and align body in straight line through shoulders to knees, push your feet firmly into wall. (Ensure the back is not arched.) Your starting point is here.

• Lift left foot from the ground and bring your knee (left) in toward the chest while keeping the hips stable (don't let them tilt or sink). Stop when the thigh is crosswise to your body while keeping the same amount of bend in knee.

• Reverse the motion to put the left foot back against the wall. That is one rep. Perform with right leg.

• Perform 10 repetitions with each leg.

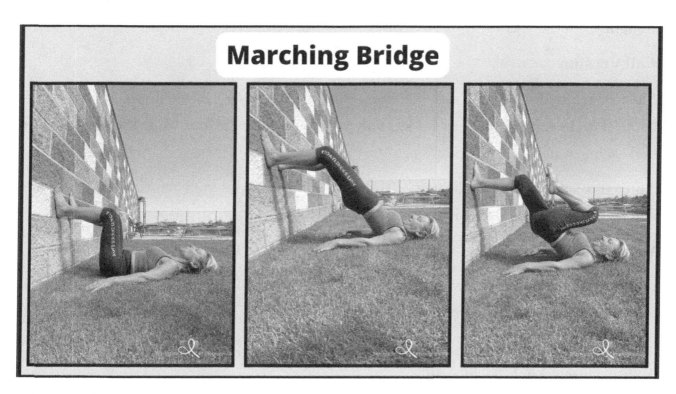

Calf raise during wall sit

• Place the back to wall as you stand. Walk with feet approximately a foot ahead before squatting down and pressing your back against wall. With the feet together, try to achieve a 90-degree bend in both the knees & hips. With palms facing one another, extend the arms in front of you at the level of your shoulders. Your starting point is here.

• While maintaining the squat stance, extend your arms in front and over your head so they come into contact with wall, and biceps next to ears.

• After bringing your arms back to the beginning position, elevate the heels off ground to perform calf raise. Your heels should touch the ground. That is one rep.

• Perform 15 repetitions.

Shoulder bridge

1: Lie on the back with knees bent & feet level on floor. The toes should contact the wall, and the feet ought to be hip-width separated. With the back on mat, visualize drawing the abdominals inward & upward.

2: Squeeze your glutes together and push the hips into air for 4 counts. Hold the position while you push into the feet for 4 counts, then roll down until 4 counts, then take a four-count break. The number of repetitions should range from four to ten, based on your degree of strength.

Wall Version

When searching for "Pilates wall exercises," this is probably what you'll see. The motion is identical to the normal shoulder bridge, only you lift & lower the hips while keeping your feet level against wall in tabletop position.

"Enter this variation with a degree of awareness that activates your hamstrings, glutes and abdominals to stabilize the spine.

Arms overhead

The chest, shoulders, & upper back may all benefit from this workout. "Those who spend their days hunched over doing their job will especially benefit from it.

1: Lean the hips, back and shoulders on the wall while facing away from it and standing with the feet approximately a foot apart.

2: Raise arms over the head, bending your elbows, and leaning back against wall while fingers contact and form shape of diamond.

3: Push the arms up, extending them as far as you're able to while keeping the fingers together as you keep elbows in touch with the wall. Six to ten times, repeat.

Wall squats

1: Stand with the feet facing out and approximately a foot farther from wall. Lean your hips, back and shoulders against wall. The palms should be towards wall, and the arms must be at the sides.

2: Slide down wall while bending your knees. Your thighs should be parallel to ground. As you perform this move, raise arms forward until they're shoulder height and parallel to floor.

3: Return your legs straight to their original positions. The arms should press back down to sides to contact wall as you perform this. You need to go down for 4 counts, retain for 4 counts, then come back up for 4 counts. Repeat six to ten times. You shouldn't keep doing it till you feel tired. Pilates does not aim to achieve that. Your quadriceps, glutes, inner thighs, hamstrings, hip flexors, back, core and shoulders will all be worked during this exercise.

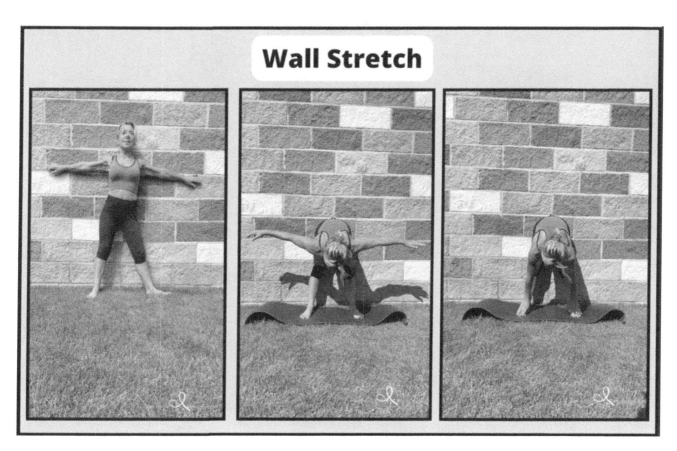

Wall Stretch

1: Lean the hips, back & shoulders against wall as you stand with the feet extended out approximately a foot & a half farther from wall.

2: Gently drop the head and pull your shoulders away from the wall, 1 vertebra at once, to start folding forward. Roll forward till just the hips are up against wall, then stop.

3: With the arms going away from the center of body, gently form five circles while positioned in this posture. 5 additional times in the other orientation, repeat this action. , then get back up using the same method, and repeat 2 to 4 times. As usual, keep the abdominals drawn in & up. There ought to be no significant strain anywhere since this activity is a stretch. Simply let your shoulders dangle and lean your low back on the wall.

2.2 Wall Poses To treat Anxiety

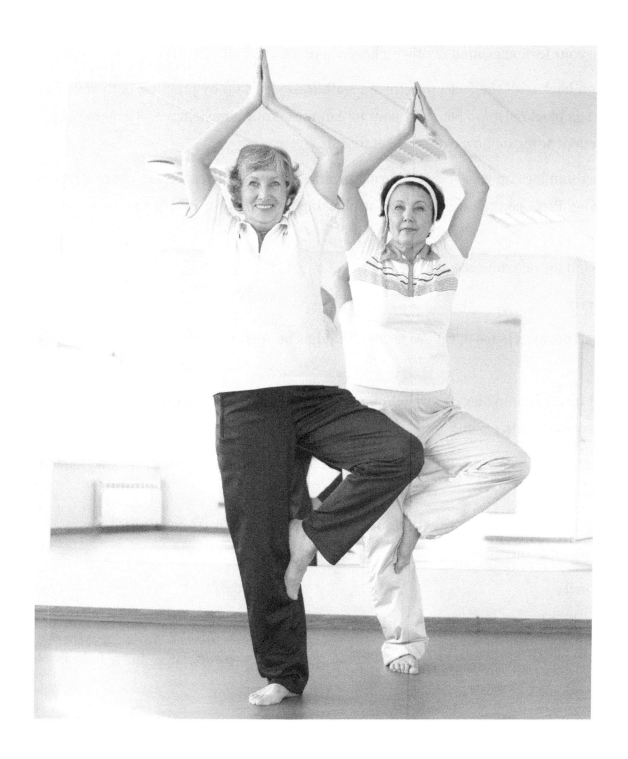

Legs Up Wall

Your mind will swiftly go from an anxious state to one of relaxation in this stance.

1. Place your feet on ground & sit with knees bent, facing wall.

2. Lie on back with the feet up against a wall. Raise hips up by pressing onto your feet, then place yoga block/cushion beneath them for support. Your hamstrings will experience a deeper stretch depending on how close you get to wall.

3. Straighten legs up wall & extend arms to sides outwards. Eyes closed, concentrate on your breathing. Practice the position without blocking beneath your hips if the lower back pain is severe.

4. Unwind for two minutes.

Butterfly

This wall position helps to relieve tension that has built up in the lower back, inner thighs, and hips.

1. Start by positioning legs on wall. You may either leave the block under or remove it to bring hips in contact with ground.

2. Kneel down and bring the feet's soles together so that they contact. Allow your knees to spread wide.

3. Rest here for a further two minutes with your arms outstretched and the eyes closed. Maintain focus on breathing.

Dragonfly

1. Begin in the previous butterfly position.

2. Next, spread your feet widely to assume a straddling stance. Feel for a holc in chest by extending arms to sides.

3. Focus on breathing for two minutes with eyes closed.

Heart Melting

A lot of us slouch over our laptops when stressed over work. The chest & shoulders will reopen in this posture, releasing any stress, tension and anxiety you may have been holding in.

1. Take a stance facing wall. Place forearms on wall while bending elbows and clasping hands.

2. Move the feet a little distance back, then drop chest toward floor while forming L shape with your hips.

3. The shoulders and chest should feel deeply stretched. For two minutes, keep your eyes closed and concentrate only on deep, deliberate breathing.

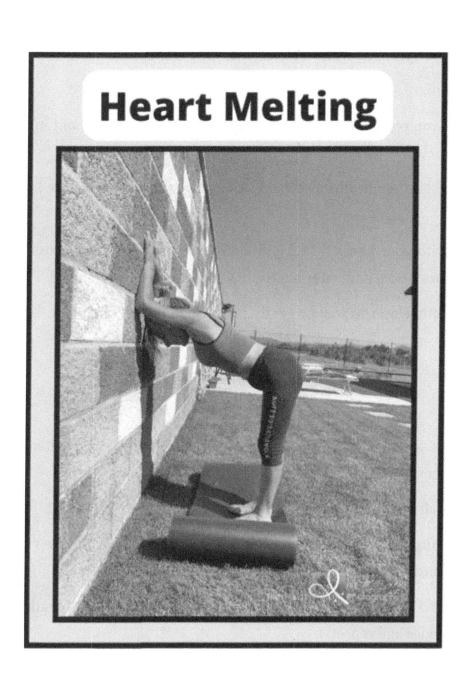

Forward Bend (Standing)

This position eases tension in hamstrings & hips while calming nervous system.

1. Place feet hip-width separated and stand up, keeping booty pressed against wall. The stretch will get deeper the closer heels are to wall.

2. Fold forward, maintaining flat back and slightly bent knees, placing hands on the floor or yoga block.

3. Spend two minutes here relaxing with your head hanging heavily.

Reclined Pigeon

This position can help you regain your calm by releasing tension that has built up in the hips & lower back.

1. Extend legs up wall while you lie down on back. About two feet from wall, the hips ought to be on ground.

2. Place feet on wall with your knees flexed and feet hip-width separated. Cross thigh (left) over the right ankle. Lower back and outer hip (right) should both feel stretched.

3. Move your hips slightly closer to wall or gently press thigh (right) open with right hand to intensify the stretch.

4. Switch legs after relaxing for two minutes with your eyes closed.

Half Dragonfly

Your hamstrings, hips & lower back will be free of any leftover stress after doing this combination of the butterfly & dragonfly postures.

1. Extend the legs up wall while lying on the back.

2. Bend left knee, moving foot to inner thigh (right), right. Following that, lower the straight leg (right) to side outwards.

3. Close the eyes, spread the arms wide to sides, and concentrate only on breathing for two minutes, then change sides and repeat.

2.3 Release Pain in Joints Using Pilates

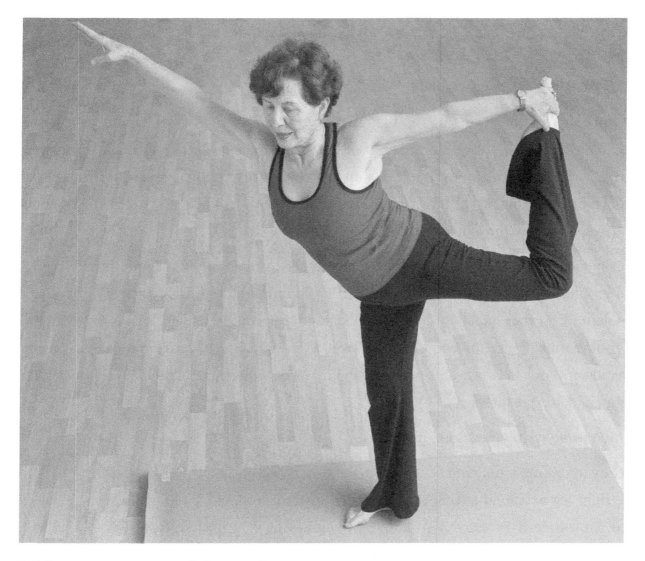

Wide-Knee Pose Involving Twist

The hip, knee, and spine may be released with the use of this stance.

1. Begin on hands & knees, forming posture of a tabletop. Widen your knees and connect your big toes. Place your hands in front as you move hips onto heels and drop chest to mat. Bring forehead to relax down. Take a minute to relax at this point by pausing.

2. To make a twist, loop right arm beneath your left while keeping your hips seated back on heels. You should place right shoulder & temple on mat. To sense stretch on inside of shoulder blade (right), slightly turn out onto right shoulder. Then take left arm and, while bending the elbow, wrap around lower back. Pause for two minutes. Return to your usual wide-knee position after putting hand (left) back down for few breaths.

3. Alternate sides, then hold for two minutes. Then relax and take a few deep breaths while holding your standard wide-knee position.

Sleeping swan

1. Get on the hands & knees in tabletop posture to start.

2. Lift right leg carefully, bringing right knee in front. Position right knee behind right wrist. Your shin ought to go across top of mat but doesn't have to be level. To safeguard knee joint, bend right toes backward toward shin. Sit up straight with your hips square in front. Take three deep breaths now. Right hip stretch should be felt. Always take a step back if it seems excessive or if you have any knee discomfort.

3. After taking three breaths, you may decide whether to maintain chest upright or lower it toward ground if you want to experience more profound stretch in right hip. If you are still able to do it, drop your hands to chest & forehead after first walking your hands forward and down to forearms. Pause for two minutes. Then raise right leg upwards and back after you walk hands upwards to lift chest & press into palms. Shake out right leg, then swap sides after regaining tabletop posture.

Shoelace pose with stretches of wrists

1. Start by assuming a tabletop stance while getting down on hands & knees. Cross knees to ensure right leg is behind left. Spread feet wide toward borders of mat while keeping knees crossed. Sit with legs traversed in front by slowly lowering your hips downwards between feet. In order to alleviate any discomfort, put a block beneath sitting bones.

2. Sit up straight by Walking hands back and flex feet to safeguard your knees. Now pause for one minute. Take note of hip stretch.

3. Next, rotate your hands over so that tops are on floor and the fingers are pointed in your direction to locate wrist stretch. To experience stretch through wrists, softly lean towards the hands. After holding for one minute, gently lift yourself to release, then swap sides.

Toe Squat

Joints in ankles, toes and plantar fascia are released in this position. This challenging stance is necessary to make sure we are mindful of our ankles & feet.

1. Get into a tabletop posture and tuck your toes.

2. Slowly drop hips onto heels by moving hands back into your legs. Ensure that toes are sufficiently tucked in so that weight is supported by balls of feet rather than your toes.

3. Ensure that pinky toes are tucked under by sitting up straight with chest out. Put hands on thighs, draw your tummy in, and concentrate on your breathing. Pause for two minutes. To conclude, untuck the toes, move hands back out to tabletop posture, and paddle tops of feet onto mat. You'll experience blood rush when it returns.

Advice: If you're unfamiliar with Pilates, this posture might feel quite unpleasant. Maintain your breathing awareness and continue to breathe through discomfort. Be mindful to leave the pose if it starts to hurt.

Fish (Supported) with Split Bridge Legs

While broken bridge posture with legs aids in releasing joints of hips & lower spine, supported fish posture helps to release tension in joints of chest & shoulders.

1. To start, arrange a single block straight at top of mat along with a block vertically down the mat, a few inches lower. The blocks need to be placed in lowest setting.

2. Sit ahead of blocks with your feet level on floor and knees bent. As you carefully lower your body onto blocks, fall back onto the hands. The head should be supported by block at top of mat, while the second block ought to be between the shoulder blades. Butt should always be on the ground.

3. Cactus the arms to ensure the palms are facing up and elbows are level with shoulders. Keep your eyes closed and take several deep breaths. Hold for three minutes.

Crossover of the right and left legs

1. Your butt should be against wall as you lie on back, your knees should be bent, and your feet should be placed three to four feet up wall. Cross right ankle on top of left knee as you lift your back and butt off the ground.

2. Pulse knee in the direction of wall twenty times without altering any other part of body. Repeat on left side after lowering your body.

Wall scissors

1. Start with feet firmly placed on wall, your knees bent, and butt near the wall. To assist lower body, raise the hips, place hands on hips, and rest your elbows on the ground.

2. Move feet up wall so your legs straighten. Your starting point is here.

From here, while maintaining both legs erect, drop left leg towards head. Repeat using right after moving left leg to beginning position. Alternate until you have done all reps.

Upward Bound

1. With your legs bent, lie on back with feet up against a wall. Put your hips in the bridge position by lifting them off ground.

2. Begin by assuming a bridge stance, then walk feet up & back down. So, alternate between straightening and bending your legs. And shift the leg up & down.

3. keep hips up throughout and bend.

4. Perform ten repetitions for each leg

One-legged bridge

1. Stand with your butt about one foot from wall. Start by hanging your right leg up in air while placing other leg on wall.

2. With your left leg bent, push the hip up five times. Then swap feet, but refrain from letting your hip drop down. Repeat 5 times as well.

Wall sit

1. Place weight on heels of feet and lean back against wall with your butt and tailbone against wall. You should have the ability to lift your toes and wiggle them.

2. Position legs at an angle of 90 degrees. If you cannot feel this posture in your hamstrings, you're probably pushing into toes rather than your heels.

3. As strongly as you are able to, press back onto wall and into heels. Hold the posture for as much time as you are able to.

Wall lunge

1. To begin, place leg (left) on floor and your right leg against a wall. As you lower yourself into squat, keep a sufficient distance from wall so that the knee does not go over toe.

2. As a result, you are approaching straight down, up, down, & up. Do five repetitions on one leg, then switch legs and repeat.

Bridges with Single Leg

1. This exercise will help you tone your glutes and hamstrings. Your feet should be up against wall while you lie on ground.

2. Aim to keep your feet flat on the wall & not lower than knee. With knee still bent slightly, raise a single foot off wall. As you raise your hips equally into air, contract your glutes.

3. Do this activity with the two feet on wall if you're having trouble maintaining hips square. Perform fifteen to twenty reps on one leg.

Windshield wipers

1. Develop your core while trimming your waist. Your legs should be up against wall while you lie on ground.

2. Utilizing your core, carefully drop legs to 1 side of wall while squeezing legs together. As legs descend, the hip on the other side will rise off the floor. When you can twist your spine the most without losing abdominal engagement, move legs up wall to middle by pulling your abs in even further.

3. Lower the opposite side's legs gradually. 10 times in each direction, repeat.

Knee stretches (Incline)

1. With this motion, you may build powerful abs, arms, & shoulders. Put both feet up on wall at back and get into incline position for push up.

2. Your hips will be just a little bit lower than your legs. Pull a single knee into chest using abdominals without moving upper body, then gently straighten leg to put foot back against the wall.

3. Perform ten repetitions on each side.

Control Balance

1. When performed against a wall, this classic Pilates movement is more difficult. The exercise's name should be sufficient to tell. It's a matter of balance & control! The wall may be used to exercise shoulders and arms as well.

2. As though you were about to do a handstand, position yourself. Walk the legs up wall while keeping hands on floor so that they are level to floor. The angle between legs & torso should be 90 degrees.

3. As far up you possibly can without lifting the foot off the wall, steadily straighten a leg up towards ceiling while maintaining control.

4. Repeat on other side, gradually lowering first leg back to wall. Perform three times for each leg.

Wall Sit employing Arm Circles

1. The quadriceps, back, & arms are toned with this workout. Squat down while keeping back against wall to target the quadriceps. It's also a great idea to lean against wall to improve your posture.

2. Pulling navel towards your back, seek to flatten whole spine on wall in this posture. Your quads will receive more of workout the deeper you squat.

3. Soften knees slightly to flatten the back against wall, making the movement more of back & arms workout. If you have light weights, you can employ them for this workout. 4. Raise the arms upward until knuckles hit the wall, palms facing wall. Do not elevate your shoulders.

5. Circle arms down and around by sides slowly. Rotate palms downward towards wall & repeat three times before turning around and going the other way.

2.4 Resistance Bands and Pilates

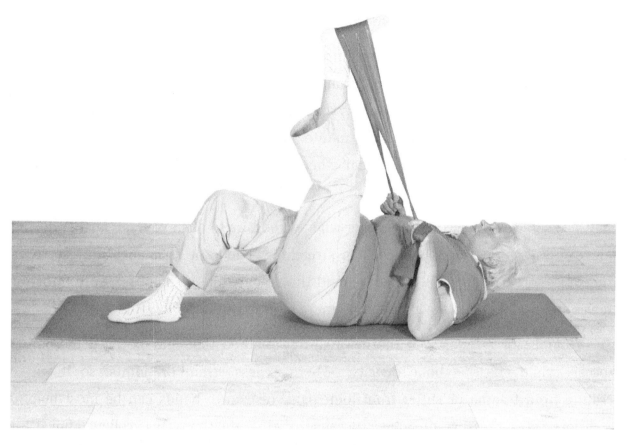

How to decide which resistance band is best for you

Resistance bands are available in a wide variety of configurations and may be used for a wide variety of sorts of exercises. Some of the more common applications for resistance bands include physical therapy, prior to exercising mobility warmups, muscle building, agility and speed drills, & stretching. You have a few options to select from when it comes to the kinds of bands for resistance that you may use based on the exercises that you want to do. Some of them have the appearance of a long, circular tube having handles on both ends, while others have the appearance of a smaller loop that is closed up at one end. The smaller closed loop band for resistance is ideal for working out glutes, legs and lower body, while longer bands for resistance with grips may be utilized for upper body as well as full body exercises.

Because resistance bands are very affordable in comparison to machines while taking up very little room in storage, they are an excellent choice to keep on hand as a backup alternative. In addition to lifting weights and engaging in a variety of cardiovascular activities, such as swimming or walking, it is suggested to combine resistance band workouts two to three times each week.

What is the mechanism behind resistance bands?

When you utilize a band that provides resistance, the band stretches to produce tension, and the muscles need to work against this opposing force in order to get a successful workout. Doing so forces your muscles to work harder, which ultimately results in a more powerful and pronounced muscle. You can incorporate them into heavy bars for more resistance, and they'll help you increase your range of movement when weights cease to operate as a result of gravity.

They may also serve as your workout partner when you desire to push yourself farther during a certain exercise as well as stretch. When stretching, bands of resistance may serve as substitutes of another individual to help extend the reach while offering pressure. Most of their moves additionally call for a greater amount of core activation.

The use of bands for resistance is another risk-free method that may be used to combat osteoporosis while boosting bone density. "There is less strain on joints, so if you're recuperating from trauma or suffer from joint pain, resistance bands can be most helpful friends. There's less pressure on joints. Because of this, they are an excellent choice for novices. Resistance bands are adaptable and can be utilized used to train a wide variety of muscle groups without putting undue stress on joints. Effective usage of them is possible for everyone, from novices to experienced individuals.

Bicep curl while standing

1. Place feet over the center of band while standing with feet separated by shoulder width.

2. Begin by grabbing a handle with each hand while keeping your arms at your sides.

3. Pull the arms toward the shoulders while keeping palms facing front and bend at the elbows to create a strong bicep contraction.

4. Gradually lower to starting position.

5. Perform 12 to 15 curls.

Bicep curl while standing

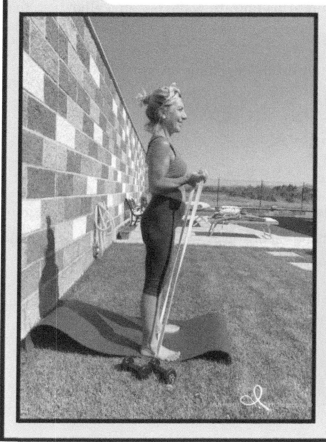 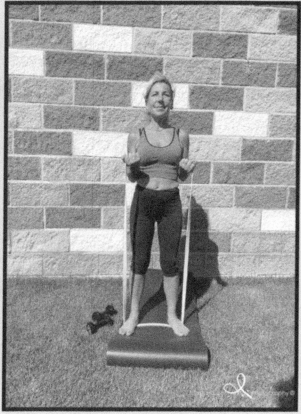

Triceps kickback

1. Place feet together and lean forward so that you are standing over the middle of band.

2. Place arms at sides with palms pointing behind you, holding one end of band in hands.

3. To get your forearms level to floor, bend your elbows while keeping them at your sides.

4. After that, Press arms completely down, moving band behind the body until arms completely extend.

5. Lower back to starting position

6. Perform 8 to 10 repetitions.

Overhead extension of triceps

1. While seated, place the tube band's middle under your glutes.

2. Holding a handle with each hand, extend your arms upward while bending elbows so that the handles are behind the neck.

3. Press the arms upward until they are completely extended, palms towards the ceiling.

4. Retract downward.

5. Perform 10 to 12 repetitions before alternating sides.

Kneeling Crunch

1. To begin, fasten the band to high anchor (this could be the highest point of cable column or door), kneel down while holding each side of band facing away from anchor, and draw band over your shoulder with your elbows bent.

2. Extend the elbows outward at shoulder height, tighten your abdominal muscles, & crunch down into your hips.

3. Take it slowly back to where you were.

4. Do this 10 to 12 times.

Russian twist

1. Wrap the band's center around the soles of your feet while seated on floor with legs fully extended.

2. With both hands, hold free ends firmly.

3. Keep your feet flat on the ground and slightly flex your knees. Then, lean back at an angle of 45 degrees.

4. Rotate band to the right by placing right hand by right hip downwards and left hand over your body.

5. While maintaining neutral posture in your midsection & low back, pull band toward right hip by contracting the oblique muscles.

6. Go back to the beginning position.

7. Perform 10–12 repetitions on each side.

Bent-over row

1. Place your feet separated by shoulder width & stand over middle of the band.

2. Keep hips in a backward position and bend the knees slightly.

3. Place your hands on outsides of knees & grasp band handles.

4. Pull band upwards into hips while bending elbows and pushing shoulder blades tight until elbows are at an angle of 90 degrees.

5. Lower, then row for ten to twelve repetitions.

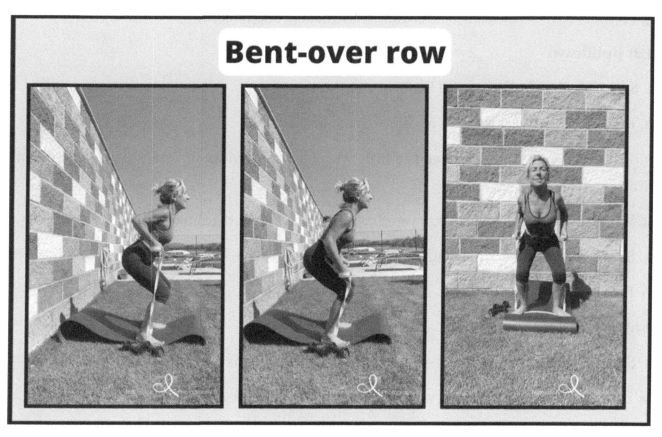

Seated row

1. With your arms outstretched and palms towards each other, grasp the band using both hands.

2. Pull band into your core while sitting up straight, bending at elbows and pulling shoulder blades tight. If it could assist you in sitting upright, feel free to gently bend the knees.

3. Take it slowly back to beginning position.

4. Perform 10–12 repetitions.

Pull apart

1. Stand with feet separated by shoulder width and the knees bent slightly.

2. Hold the center of band firmly in both palms, with your shoulders as your distance between your hands, at level of shoulders and palms pointing down.

3. While maintaining straight arm position, pull band out & back until the shoulder blades tighten.

4. Take it slowly back to beginning position.

5. Perform 8–10 repetitions of stretching, contracting, and releasing.

Lat pulldown

1. Secure the band to horizontal bar over your head.

2. Kneel with your face towards anchor so band is in front.

3. Hold each end using your hands a little wider than the width of your shoulders and your arms stretched above.

4. While tightening the muscles in your back, pull band toward ground while bending elbows.

5. Slowly lift hands back to beginning position once they have reached shoulders.

6. Perform 10–12 repetitions.

Lateral raise

1. Stand with your feet shoulder-width apart and above the middle of a tube band.

2. Hold onto each handle using your hands facing in and your arms at sides.

3. Extend the arms out to sides to level of shoulder while gently bending elbows.

4. Slowly go back down.

5. Aim for 8 to 10 reps.

Upright row

1. With the feet separated by shoulder width and above the band's middle, grab handles with palms facing you and place them close to front of thighs.

2. With elbows bent & in high V posture, draw band upwards from front of body to level of shoulders.

3. Retract your steps back to beginning point.

4. Continue rowing for ten to twelve repetitions.

Deadlift with a single leg Using Dumbbells

1. Place one hand on wall while holding the dumbbell in the other hand.

2. Raise closest leg to wall off ground & bend hip and knee on the leg that is grounded.

3. Keep your back straight and your lower back in arch as you hinge at hips.

4. Go back to the beginning position whenever you feel pull in hamstring.

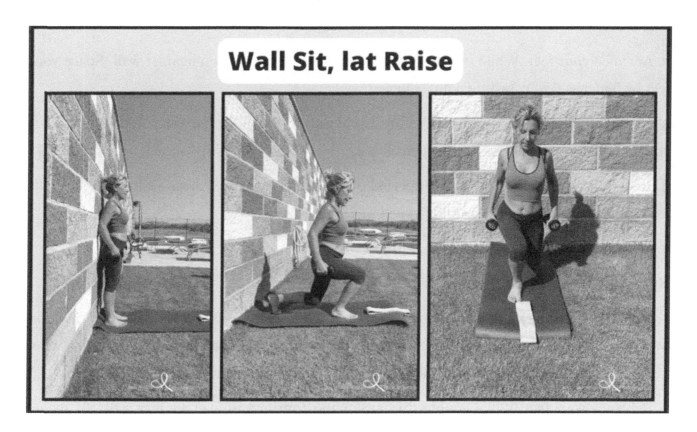

Wall Sit, Lat Raise

1. Stand with feet separated by shoulder width and rest against wall with feet securely rooted in ground. With palms facing body, hold dumbbells by your sides. Keep your core engaged and the elbows bent slightly.

2. Advance your feet. As you're doing, stoop and continue to lean against wall. Seperate feet by six inches. Your starting point is here.

3. After exhaling, gently lower yourself into the ideal wall sit posture. Raise the arms until they're level to floor & level with shoulders.

4. After a little period of holding this posture, inhale and move up while straightening the arms. Lower the arms and return to your beginning posture at the same time.

5. Perform three 10-rep sets.

Wall Sit Curls

1. Stand with feet separated by shoulder width and lean onto wall with feet planted in ground. With palms pointing forward, elbows close to body, and core tightened, hold dumbbells at your sides.

2. Advance your feet. While you do this, stoop and continue to lean against wall. Space your feet by 6 inches. Your starting point is here.

3. Next, let out a breath and lower yourself into an ideal wall sits posture. Keep upper arms still, bend elbows, and raise both of your forearms until dumbbells are almost near shoulders.

4. Remain in this posture for a brief period of time, then exhale & move wall. Straighten the arms while simultaneously lowering your forearms.

5. Perform two to three sets of 10 repetitions.

Shoulder Press with Wall sit

1. Stand with feet separated by shoulder width and lean onto wall with feet planted on floor. With the palms of your hands facing forward and arms at an angle of 90 degrees to forearms, hold dumbbells while flexing your elbows so that upper arms are level with shoulders.

2. Advance your feet. While you do this, stoop and continue to lean against wall. Six inches should separate your feet. Your starting point is here.

3. After that, exhale & slide to wall sit posture. Raise the arms simultaneously so that they're straight over your head and completely stretched.

4. Remain in this posture for a moment.

5. Take a deep breath in, flex the elbows, bring your arms down, slide upward while resting on wall, and return to the beginning position.

Wall Sit with Straight Leg Raise

1. Stand with feet separated by shoulder width and rest against wall with feet planted in floor.

2. Advance your feet. When you do this, stoop and continue to lean against wall. Space feet apart by 6 inches. Your starting point is here.

3. Move down to wall sit posture.

4. Straighten right leg in front of you.

5. Keep this position for five seconds.

6. Breathe in and drop your leg gradually.

7. Maintain your balance when sitting.

8. After exhaling, do the same with your left leg.

9. Perform one 10-rep session.

Wall Sit, Including Marching

1. Stand shoulder-width apart and lean against the wall with your feet firmly planted in the ground.

2. Step forward and lower yourself as you do so. Place your feet 6 inches apart and continue to lean on the wall. Your starting point is here.

3. Climb down to a wall-sitting posture and relax.

4. As you exhale, raise your right and left legs to your chest in a marching motion.

5. Perform three 10-rep sets.

With Heel Lift, Wall Sit

1. Stand with feet separated by shoulder width and rest against wall with feet planted in floor.

2. Step forward and lower yourself as you do so. Place your feet 6 inches apart and continue to lean on the wall. Your starting point is here.

3. Move down to a chair or wall sit posture, and tighten your abdominal muscles.

4. Raise both of your heels, then pause for 5 to 10 seconds.

5. Let go of the hold, lower heels & repeat.

6. Perform two 10-rep sets.

Resistance Band Wall Sit

1. Wrap your thighs with resistance band.

2. Stand with feet separated by shoulder width and rest against wall with feet planted in floor.

3. Step forward and lower yourself as you do so. Place your feet 6 inches apart and continue to lean on the wall. Your starting point is here.

4. Next, lower yourself to sitting posture while spreading your legs apart.

5. Reverse your motion and return to the starting position.

6. Do two sets of ten repetitions.

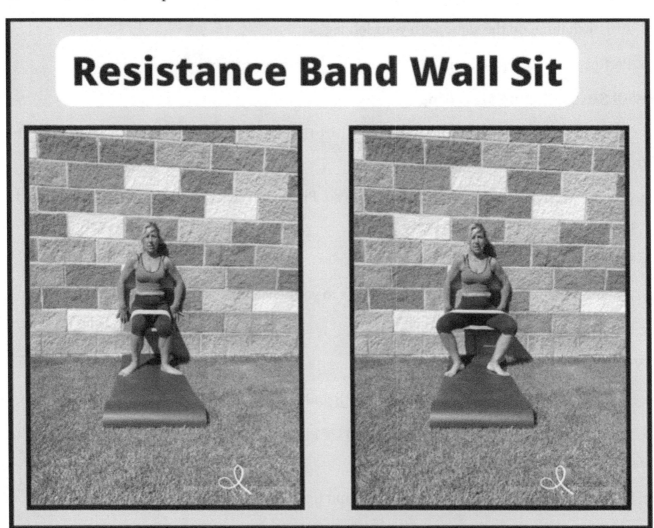

Wall Sit incorporating Medicine Ball

1. Stand with feet separated by shoulder width and rest against wall with feet planted in floor.

2. Step forward and lower yourself as you do so. Place your feet 6 inches apart and continue to lean on the wall. Your starting point is here.

3. Squeeze medicine ball while lowering yourself gradually.

4. Remain in this posture for brief moment before returning to the beginning position.

5. Perform two ten-rep sets.

Crossed Arms Wall sit

1. Leaning on the wall first. Keep feet planted on ground, separated at shoulder width.

2. Step forward and descend a bit. Spread your feet apart 6 inches. Keep your arms crossed and close to chest level. Your starting point is here.

3. Next, slide down slowly and maintain the chair posture for ten seconds.

4. After exhaling, rise to your initial posture.

5. Perform two ten-rep sets.

Wall sit incorporating Stability Ball

1. Put a stability ball between you and wall. Maintain feet planted on ground and separated by shoulder width.

2. Step forward & descend a bit. Make sure the feet are spaced six inches apart.

3. You have a choice of using resistance band or doing bicep curl and shoulder press. As you slowly descend, keep stability ball balanced to prevent it from slipping and falling.

4. After holding the chair posture for ten seconds, return to the beginning position.

Chapter 3: 21-Day Workout Plan

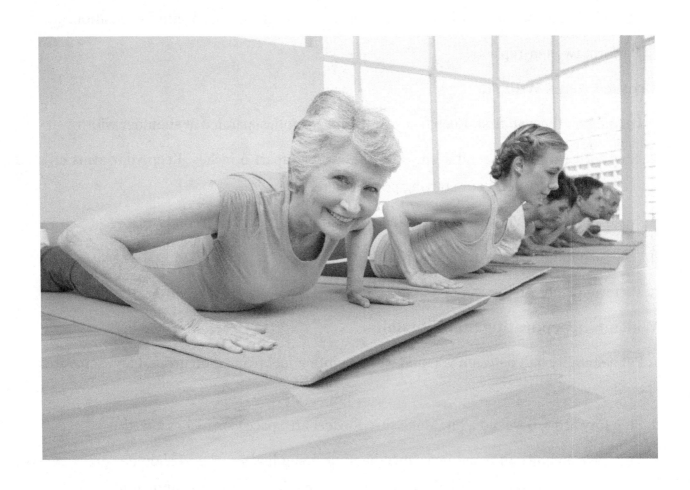

Week 1

Day 1	Warm Up	Main Workout	Cool Down
	Spinal Twist	Triceps kickback	Cobra
	Cat stretch	Overhead extension of triceps	Arm reach & pull
	Head Nod	Kneeling Crunch	
	Spinal Twist	Russian twist	
Day 2	Warm Up	Main Workout	Cool Down
	Cobra	Bent-over row	Pelvic Thrust
	Downward Pilates wall rolls	Seated row	Stretch of spine
	Spinal Twist	Pull apart	
	Shoulder bridge	Lat pulldown	
	Head Nod		
Day 3	Warm Up	Main Workout	Cool Down
	Cat stretch	Lateral raise	Spinal Twist
	Swan prep	Upright row	Head Nod
	Stretch of spine	Deadlift with a single leg Using Dumbbells	
	Spinal Twist	Wall Sit, Lat Raise	

Day 4	Warm Up	Main Workout	Cool Down
	Arm reach & pull	Wall Sit Curls	Arm reach & pull
	Cobra	Shoulder Press with Wall sit	Butterfly Stretch
	Cat stretch	Wall Sit with Straight Leg Raise	
	Spinal Twist	Wall Sit, Including Marching	
Day 5	Warm Up	Main Workout	Cool Down
	Head Nod	With Heel Lift, Wall Sit	Pilates Imprinting
	Pelvic Thrust	Resistance Band Wall Sit	Swan prep
	Stretch of spine	Wall Sit incorporating Medicine Ball	
	Cobra	Crossed Arms Wall sit	
Day 6	Warm Up	Main Workout	Cool Down
	Downward Pilates wall rolls	Wall sit incorporating Stability Ball	Arm reach & pull
	Head Nod	Chest opener	Pelvic Thrust
	Spinal Twist	Wall sits	
	Cat stretch	Deadlift with a single leg Using Dumbbells	

Day 7	Warm Up	Main Workout	Cool Down
	Assisted Roll down	Supported Half Lunge	Arm reach & pull
	Hip opener (Standing)	Knee Raise (Standing)	Butterfly Stretch
	Leg swing (Side)	Arm Raise (Wall DB)	
	Calf stretch (Active)	Arm Circles (Walls DB)	

Week 2

	Warm Up	Main Workout	Cool Down
Day 1	Spinal Twist Cat stretch Cobra Head Nod	Hip Release Hip Roll Shrug Arm Circle	Toe Tap Spine Twist (seated)
Day 2	Pilates Imprinting Arm reach & pull Pelvic Thrust Swan prep	Roll into bridge upwards Kneeling to Side with Leg Lift Side Plank, Including Rotation Quadruped Extension of Leg	Butterfly Stretch Forward fold (Seated)
Day 3	Downward Pilates wall rolls Stretch of spine Cobra Head Nod	Triceps jut out and lateral leg lift Wall roll down Semi-lunge with support Knee Crunch with Single-Leg	Toe Tap Spine Twist (seated)

	Warm Up	Main Workout	Cool Down
Day 4	Spinal Twist Cat stretch Cobra Head Nod	Calf Raise with Wall Bridge Reach Backs Marching Bridge Calf raise during wall sit	Butterfly Stretch Forward fold (Seated)
Day 5	Spinal Twist Cat stretch Cobra Head Nod	Shoulder bridge Arms overhead Wall squats Wall Stretch	Toe Tap Forward fold (Seated)
Day 6	Pilates Imprinting Arm reach & pull Pelvic Thrust Swan prep	*Legs Up Wall* Butterfly Dragonfly Heart Melting	Spine Twist (seated) Butterfly Stretch
Day 7	Downward Pilates wall rolls Head Nod Cat stretch Cobra	Forward Bend (Standing) Reclined Pigeon Half Dragonfly Shoelace pose with stretches of wrists	Pilates Imprinting Arm reach & pull

Week 3

Day 1	Warm Up	Main Workout	Cool Down
	Spinal Twist	Wide-Knee Pose Involving Twist	Pelvic Thrust
	Cat stretch	Sleeping swan	Swan prep
	Cobra	Toe Squat	
	Head Nod	Fish (Supported) with Split Bridge Legs	
Day 2	Warm Up	Main Workout	Cool Down
	Pilates Imprinting	Crossover of the right and left legs	Downward Pilates wall rolls
	Arm reach & pull	Wall scissors	Stretch of spine
	Pelvic Thrust	Upward Bound	
	Swan prep	One-legged bridge	
Day 3	Warm Up	Main Workout	Cool Down
	Downward Pilates wall rolls	Wall sit	Toe Tap
	Stretch of spine	Wall lunge	Spine Twist (seated)
	Cobra	Bridges with Single Leg	
	Head Nod	Bicep curl while standing	

Day 4	**Warm Up**	**Main Workout**	**Cool Down**
	Spinal Twist	Forward Bend (Standing)	Forward fold (Seated)
	Cat stretch	Reclined Pigeon	Stretch of spine
	Cobra	Sleeping swan	
	Head Nod	Toe Squat	
Day 5	**Warm Up**	**Main Workout**	**Cool Down**
	Pilates Imprinting	Kneeling to Side with Leg Lift	Butterfly Stretch
	Arm reach & pull	Side Plank, Including Rotation	Downward Pilates wall rolls
	Swan prep	Triceps jut out and lateral leg lift	
	Cobra	Wall roll down	
Day 6	**Warm Up**	**Main Workout**	**Cool Down**
	Cobra	Hip Roll	Pilates Imprinting
	Cat stretch	Shrug	Swan prep
	Head Nod	Quadruped Extension of Leg	
	Pelvic Thrust	Semi-lunge with support	
Day 7	**Warm Up**	**Main Workout**	**Cool Down**
	Downward Pilates wall rolls	Knee Crunch with Single-Leg	Arm reach & pull
	Stretch of spine	Reach Backs	Pelvic Thrust
	Cobra	Arms overhead	
	Head Nod	Butterfly	

Conclusion

Pilates has quickly become the exercise of choice for a variety of reasons, including better flexibility and strength, reduced risk of injury, and rehabilitation. According to the findings of a recent survey, gym-goers in UK are more likely to participate in pilates over yoga these days.

Pilates has had a remarkable impact on both my physical conditioning and overall health. And it ought to alter yours as well; Joseph Pilates remained physically fit even into his eighties as a direct result of this exercise routine. An individual interested in becoming a Pilates learner has access to a wide variety of class choices. Pilates classes geared at older adults are a fantastic way to maintain flexibility, alleviate aches & pains, and make acquaintances in social setting.

After some time spent becoming used to it, you could decide that Pilates is the new go-to form of exercise. That's fantastic...as provided that you combine your Pilates sessions with another type of physical activity each week.

It's not always an isolated exercise. The heart rate will increase since you are training different muscle groups, so be prepared for that. However, Pilates isn't as intense a cardiovascular exercise as other forms of exercise. Although it does include some intense stretching as well as some weight training, Pilates ought to continue to be an element of a well-rounded workout routine.

To put it another way, doing Pilates anywhere from up to 5 times per week is an excellent choice, but you ought to additionally make it a point to engage in activities that develop strength in your arms and shoulders, such as resistance training, plus aerobic exercise, such as cycling, on a weekly basis.

A low-impact, full-body exercise, Pilates, which has been practiced for nearly a century, is something that may be an excellent addition to fitness routine that is already well-balanced. The study on the health advantages of Pilates has produced conclusive results, and it implies that Pilates may have a favorable influence on your mental and physical well-being. Finding a qualified teacher and having a conversation with your primary

care provider can assist you in determining the entry point that is both the safest & most productive for you. From afar, it may seem to be frightening.

You've probably battled through glute bridges as well as the iconic Pilates maneuver known as hundred if you've tried any kind of Pilates before. Both of these exercises help strengthen your core. You are now a Wall Pilates gal if, instead of using a band, ball or reformer equipment to execute the exercises, you use the wall as prop. Wall Pilates is a modification of mat Pilates in which you do exercises like the wall squats, hundred and plank while pushing several body parts (often the feet) against wall. Not only does the wall serve to give stability and balance, but it also contributes to the challenge by offering resistance. And although your buttocks and abdominal region will feel the heat from Wall Pilates routines the most, your upper body won't be left out of sweat sessions thanks to standing movements that target the arms & chest (consider wall planks and Push-ups).

Pilates is one of the few forms of exercise that offers low-impact movements that are beneficial to your mental and physical well-being (hello, body-mind connection!). You will have a difficult time finding another kind of exercise that has these features. Forget about purchasing any huge or costly pieces of exercise equipment; all you require to break a sweat is the blank wall in your room that you have wanted to decorate. The most exciting part? It won't create a dent in your pocketbook. Consider the 4 walls in living room or home office to be the sole prop that you require to get Pilates on. Whether you utilize it as additional support or a means to level up the mat practice, think of walls as sole accessory you require to get the Pilates on.

Make use of this guide as a starting point for your Pilates practice. Everyone who has given it a go has been astonished by the outcomes, particularly by the fact that such little actions may have such significant and beneficial effects on body. Having said that, when it comes to anything that has connection with your well-being, you should always spare time to do the research. Once you get started, I have no doubt that you will not be let down. I can't wait to hear that you have the same level of satisfaction with Pilates as I did! I really wish that you found this guide to be informative.

Frame here to download your BONUS

90-day Training Book to Get Everything Under Control

Review this book

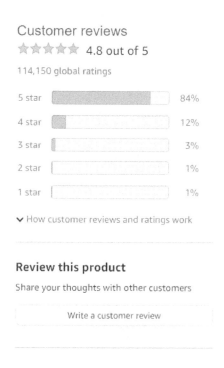

Thank you for reading this far! I would be extremely grateful if you would take a minute of your time to leave an honest review of my work on Amazon.

Made in the USA
Las Vegas, NV
07 October 2023

78717101R00063